About The Cover

A Maiden's Head

Leonardo Da Vinci (1452-1519)

Credit: Da Vinci/Alinari/Art Resource, NY

The image is believed by scholars to be a portrait of one of the first female physicians. Her humble, healing glance seems to embody the culture of sincere humanism that exists amongst the physician-leaders featured in these pages.

We are incredibly grateful for the support we received from The Honorable Akila Kridene and Sophie Nadea at United States Embassy Paris, Ms. Croisine Martin-Roland at Musée du Louvre, and Mr. Robbi Siegel at Art Resource in New York. We express our gratitude for their generosity in sharing the rights to this piece for the cover.

D1455930

Introduction

The Service Minded Physician is a medical textbook on becoming a leader in alleviating suffering for the medically underserved.

Far from a comprehensive clinical field manual, we intend for this to be a compass of human relationships for a medical student or physician trainee, providing him or her certain tools. These include the humility, courage, and audacity necessary to build relationships with those who have been disadvantaged by society and to dedicate a portion of his or her life in medicine to becoming an innovator for uplifting the medically underserved.

We believe that groundbreaking leadership requires groundbreaking mentorship. As discovery in academic medicine evolves at a record pace, coupled with increasing clinical care needs, a U.S. physician-leader's time is often limited. We thus present to you a few half-pieces of paper with the dedication of our worlds' physician-leaders who pursue health equity on a daily basis in a format mirroring the kind of conversation you might have on an airplane.

Nobel Laureate Albert Camus shared his thoughts on mentorship:
"Don't walk in front of me, I may not follow;
Don't walk behind me, I may not lead;
Walk beside me, and just be my friend."

We hope to provide an opportunity for current medical students and trainees to walk beside our generation's Albert Schweitzer's. We created an interview template with the intention of providing the next physician-leaders with viewpoints on the patient-doctor relationship that are equally comprehensive and diverse: with the ubiquitous intention of probing your own reflection on the pursuit of health equity.

Inspired by the concise yet direct themed-pedagogy of Facebook, Twitter, and Instagram comments with which our generation was raised, we elected to use a phrase-question pair interview template. Beginning with an inquiry into each physician-leader's motivations for making a larger contribution to society, and ending with an inquiry into his or her motivations for making a meaningful impact each day beneath his or her white coat, we seek to share the presence of our nation's physician-leaders.

Editors' Note: Physician-leaders were not required to respond to all phrase-question pairs or in any particular order.

Phrase-Question Pairs:

our white coat - As a physician engaged in public service, and in a leadership role, how do you believe that the white coat metaphorically belongs to both patient and doctor? At your practice's core, how are you and your patients both healers?

a story - What is your favorite story from your life in medicine, which if someone had read it to you on your first day of medical school, it would have inspired you?

attending to the world - In what ways do you believe being an attending physician in the public service inherently means serving people of all backgrounds? Feel free to share inspiring stories from your career.

uplifting the medically underserved - Is access to a physician a fundamental human right? To what extent do you view yourself, and your career, as having a role in health equity in the United States?

a life apart - As a physician-leader, when is it appropriate to feel saddened, and what are your tools for moving forward professionally in your practice? Is it appropriate to show emotion in front of your medical team and trainees?

a loving smile - As a physician, is it appropriate to bond with your patients, and in what ways do you balance personal relationships with professionalism as a leader?

a lens into your life - What is one of your best days like as a physician-leader in the public service? Physician-leaders were invited to share an inspiring photo using medicine in a public service setting, and if they elected to share such an image, it was used as their chapter's cover image.

The Service Minded Physician is arranged into four sections: *U.S. National Physician-Leaders, Health System and Medical School Leaders, Faculty and Community Leaders, and Resident and Student Leaders.* Each section is divided into chapters, with each comprising a personal interview with a physician-leader or medical student-leader. To briefly introduce the prose, our intention is to provide our medical student and trainee audience with as close to the feeling of meeting each of these people as possible. We have thus elected to present physician responses in a spoken word format with minimal edits, as opposed to more didactically revised text. Each section is curated in alphabetical order, by first name, in line with our intention to make medicine more personal.

We would like to dedicate *The Service Minded Physician* to Rachel Naomi Remen M.D. and Paul Farmer M.D. Dr. Remen thank you for having the courage to remind the world that we are each patients too, and Dr. Farmer thank you for having the courage to remind the world that life itself matters.

Editorial Team

The Service Minded Physician editorial team is comprised of faculty, residents, and students from the University of California, Los Angeles, University of California, San Francisco, and Baylor College of Medicine.

Matthew A. Rosenstein

UCLA Undergraduate Class of 2013, Duke Medical School Class of 2018

Jamie L. Yao

UCLA Undergraduate Class of 2012, UCSF School of Medicine Class of 2017

Editors-in-Chief

Isaac Yang M.D.

UCLA Assistant Professor of Neurosurgery

Daniel T. Nagasawa M.D.

Neurosurgeon, UCLA Medical Center

Physicians-in-Chief

Kristy L. Hamilton

Baylor College of Medicine Class of 2014, Medical School Class President

Christina Fong

UCLA School of Medicine Class of 2016

Amol Agarwal

University of Pennsylvania Perelman School of Medicine, Medical School Class President

Winward Choy

UCLA School of Medicine Class of 2015

Marko Spasic

UCLA School of Medicine Class of 2015

 Christine K. Thang

UCLA School of Medicine Class of 2015

Ariel Moradzadeh

Charles R. Drew University/UCLA Medical School Class of 2015

Kimberly Thill

Director, UCLA Isaac Yang Research Lab, Gonda Center

Brittany Voth

UCLA Undergraduate Class of 2014

Editors

Table Of Contents

1) U.S. National Physician-Leaders

Ardis D. Hoven, M.D., Professor of Medicine, Interim Chief, Division of Infectious Diseases, University of Kentucky. President of the American Medical Association.

Darrell G. Kirch, M.D., President and chief executive officer of the Association of American Medical Colleges (AAMC).

Deane E. Marchbein, M.D., Department of Anesthesia, Critical Care and Pain Medicine, Massachusetts General Hospital. President of Doctors Without Borders.

Francis S. Collins, M.D., Ph.D., Director of the National Institutes of Health (NIH). As a physician-geneticist, Dr. Collins served as Director of the National Human Genome Research Institute (NHGRI).

Harvey Fineberg M.D., Ph.D., President of the Institute of Medicine, Provost Emeritus of Harvard University, and Dean Emeritus of the Harvard School of Public Health and Partners Healthcare.

Joanne Liu M.D., International President of Médecins Sans Frontières (MSF), the umbrella organization of Doctors Without Borders.

Kristen DeStigter M.D., John P. and Kathryn H. Tampas Green and Gold Professor and Vice Chair of Radiology at the University of Vermont College of Medicine. Dr. DeStigter is Founder of Imaging the World.

Molly Cooke M.D., Professor of Medicine at the UCSF School of Medicine. President of the American College of Physicians and Inaugural Director of Education in Global Health Sciences at UCSF.

Paul Farmer M.D., Co-Founder of Partners in health, Kolokotrones University Professor at Harvard University, and Chief of the Division of Global Health Equity at Brigham and Woman's Hospital in Boston, Massachusetts.

Sir Richard Thompson D.M., President of the Royal College of Physicians in London. In his clinical research laboratory, he has studied various aspects of nutritional gastroenterology and published over 200 papers. He served as physician to HM The Queen for 21 years.

Thomas Frieden M.D., MPH, Director of the U.S. Centers for Disease Control and Prevention. He is trained in Internal Medicine, Infectious Diseases, Public Health, and Epidemiology.

2) Health System and Medical School Leaders

Anthony Atala M.D., W.H. Boyce Professor and Director of the Wake Forest Institute for Regenerative Medicine, and Chair of the Department of Urology at the Wake Forest School of Medicine in North Carolina. Dr. Atala developed the first lab-grown organ to be implanted into a human.

Charles Sorenson M.D., Adjust Professor of Surgery at the University of Utah, board-certified Urologic surgeon. He is President and CEO of Intermountain Healthcare.

Donna M. Ferriero M.D., W.H. and Marie Wattis Distinguished Professor & Chair of the UCSF Department of Pediatrics, and Physician-in-Chief of UCSF Benioff Children's Hospital.

Edward Benz M.D., Richard and Susan Smith Professor of Medicine, Professor of Pediatrics, Professor of Pathology and faculty Dean of Oncology at Harvard Medical School. He currently serves as President and CEO of the Dana-Farber/ Partners CancerCare, Director of the Dana-Farber Cancer Center and trustee of the Dana-Farber/Children's Hospital Cancer Care at Harvard Medical School.

Erika Goldstein, M.D., MPH,, Professor, Department of Medicine, and Associate Dean for the Colleges, University of Washington School of Medicine.

Eric Klein M.D., Chairman at the Glickman Urological & Kidney Institute and staff member in the Taussig Cancer Institute at the Cleveland Clinic.

A. Eugene Washington M.D. is Dean of the David Geffen School of Medicine and Vice Chancellor for Health Sciences at the University of California, Los Angeles. He currently leads the National Institutes of Health PCORI initiative for the medically underserved.

Gary Gottlieb M.D., MBA, Professor of Psychiatry at Harvard Medical School. He is President and CEO of Partners Healthcare, a collegium of the Harvard Medical School teaching hospitals.

Jerris Hedges, M.D., is an emergency medicine physician and Dean of the John A. Burns School of Medicine at the University of Hawaii. He serves as a member of the United States National Academies of Science Institute of Medicine and has co-authored Roberts and Hedges' Clinical Procedures in Emergency Medicine.

Jimmy Hara M.D. is Professor of Family Medicine and Associate Dean at Charles R. Drew University of Medicine and Science. He is Professor of Clinical Medicine at the David Geffen School of Medicine at UCLA. He is Credentials Chair of the American Board of Family Physicians, and currently the Los Angeles City Fire Commissioner.

John F. McGeehan M.D., FACP is Associate Dean for Student Affairs and Admissions at the Cooper Medical School of Rowan University.

Josh Adler M.D., Chief Medical Officer of UCSF Medical Center and UCSF Benioff Children's Hospital and Medical Director of UCSF Ambulatory Care.

Laurie H. Glimcher, M.D., Immunologist, Professor of Medicine, and Stephen and Suzanne Weiss Dean at Weill Cornell Medical College.

Michael V. Drake, M.D., former Chancellor of the University of California, Irvine, and Professor of Opthalmology at the University of California, Irvine School of Medicine; and currently serves as President of The Ohio State University.

Michelle Forcier M.D., Assistant Dean for Medical Education and Associate Professor of Pediatrics at the Alpert Medical School of Brown University. She is considered by many to be the nation's expert on transgender medicine.

Millard Collins M.D., Associate Professor of Family Medicine and Associate Dean for Student Affairs at Meharry Medical College.

Pascal Goldschmidt M.D., Cardiologist and cardiovascular researcher who serves as Senior Vice President for Medical Affairs and Dean of the University of Miami Leonard M. Miller School of Medicine. He is the Chief Executive Officer of the University of Miami Health System.

Paul B. Roth M.D., Chancellor for Health Sciences and Chief Executive Officer of the University of New Mexico Health System and Dean of the University of New Mexico School of Medicine. He is trained in Emergency Medicine.

Philip A. Pizzo M.D. Former Dean and the David and Susan Heckerman Professor of Pediatrics and of Microbiology and Immunology, at Stanford University School of Medicine.

Robert Grant M.D., MPH, Professor of Medicine at UCSF and Director of the Gladstone-UCSF Laboratory of Clinical Virology and Associate Director of the UCSF Center for AIDS Research. He was one of the 2012 Time Magazine 100 Most Influential People in the World: #20, Most Influential Physician.

Victor J. Dzau, M.D., James B. Duke Professor of Medicine, president and Chief Executive Officer of Duke University Health System, and Chancellor of Health Affairs at Duke University.

Wiley Souba, M.D., ScD, MBA, Professor of Surgery and Vice-President for Health Affairs and Dean of the Geisel School of Medicine at Dartmouth.

William R. Brody M.D., Ph.D., Radiologist and physician-scientist and Irwin M. Jacobs Presidential Chair and President of the Salk Institute for Biological Sciences.

3) <u>Faculty and Community Leaders</u>

Andru Ziwasimon-Zeller, M.D., Co-Founder of the Casa de Salud Medical Office in Albuquerque, New Mexico, a clinic geared towards serving low-income and uninsured patients. He is also a National Robert Wood Johnson Community Health Leader award winner.

Amy Rezak, M.D., Captain of Trauma Surgery for the United States Army and an Assistant Professor of Surgery at the University of North Carolina School of Medicine.

Arnold P. Gold, M.D., Professor of Clinical Neurology and Pediatric Neurology at Columbia University College of Physicians and Surgeons. The Arnold P. Gold Foundation, a not-for-profit whose mission is to "perpetuate the tradition of the caring doctor," is named in his honor.

Atilla Under M.D., Associate Professor of Emergency Medicine at the David Geffen School of Medicine at UCLA, Associate Medical Director at the UCLA Center for Prehospital Care. He is the Tactical Medicine Physician for the Hawthorne Police Department and Medical Team Manager, FEMA Urban Search and Rescue California Task Force 2.

Bernie Siegel M.D., Professor Emeritus in the Department of Surgery at Yale University School of Medicine and author of the New York Times #1 Bestselling Book, Love, Medicine, and Miracles.

Christine Montrossl M.D., Assistant Professor of Psychiatry and Human Behavior, Brown University School of Medicine and Bestselling Author, Body of Work.

David Wofsy M.D., Professor of Medicine and Associate Dean for Admissions at the UCSF School of Medicine. He is Past President of the American College of Rheumatology and an attending physician at San Francisco VA Medical Center.

Daniel Lowenstein M.D., Professor and Vice Chair of the Department of Neurology at UCSF Medical Center and also serves as the Director of the UCSF Epilepsy Center.

Dean Ornish M.D., Clinical Professor of Medicine at UCSF and Founder and President of the Preventative Medicine Research Institute. He is the author of six best-selling books including The Spectrum, and personal physician to President Bill Clinton and Secretary of State Hillary Rodham Clinton.

Dean Schillinger M.D., Professor of Medicine and Chief of the UCSF Division of General Internal Medicine at the San Francisco General Hospital (SFGH) and Trauma Center. He is also the Director of the Health Communications Program at the UCSF Center for Vulnerable Populations.

Ellen Beck, M.D., Clinical Professor of Family and Preventive Medicine at the UCSD School of Medicine, founding Director of the Student Run Free Clinic Project, Director of Medical Student Education for the Division of Family Medicine, and Director of Education for the new Center for Integrative Medicine at the University of California, San Diego.

Fabien Koskas, M.D., Professor and Chief of Vascular Surgery at Pitié-Salpêtrière University Hospital in Paris, France.

Isaac Yang, M.D., Assistant Professor of Neurosurgery at the David Geffen School of Medicine at UCLA and a principal investigator in the UCLA Malignant Brain Tumor Laboratory.

Josh Broder M.D., Associate Professor of Surgery, Division of Emergency Medicine at Duke University School of Medicine. He also serves as the Duke University Emergency Medicine Residency Program Director.

Linda Regan M.D., Assistant Professor and Program Director at the Johns Hopkins Emergency Medicine Residency. She also serves as Director of the Medical Education Fellowship.

Lloyd Michener M.D., Professor of Community and Family Medicine, Clinical Professor in the School of Nursing, and Chair of the Department of Community and Family Medicine at Duke University School of Medicine.

Louise Aronson M.D., Associate Professor of Geriatrics at UCSF. Recipient of the Arnold P. Gold Foundation Gold Professorship and author of A History of the Present Illness.

Martin A. Finkel, D.O., Professor of Pediatrics, Founder and Medical Director of the Child Abuse Research Education and Service (CARES) Institute at the Rowan University School of Osteopathic Medicine.

Mayer B. Davidson M.D., Professor of Medicine at the Charles R. Drew University of Medicine and Science, Professor of Medicine at the David Geffen School of Medicine at UCLA, Co-Founder of the Venice Family Clinic and Director of the Diabetes Program in the Martin Luther King Multi-service Ambulatory Care Center (MLK-MACC).

Michael Gisondi M.D., Associate Professor of Emergency Medicine and Emergency Medicine Residency Program Director at The Feinberg School of Medicine at Northwestern.

Pablo Hernandez-Itriago, M.D., Clinical Associate Professor in the Department of Family Medicine at the Boston University School of Medicine and serves as Medical Director at the South End Community Health Center.

Patch Adams, M.D., Founder of the Gesundheit Free Clinic in the West Virginia Mountains and the physician upon which the Academy Award-acclaimed film Patch Adams is based.

Rachel Naomi Remen, M.D., Clinical Professor of Family and Community Medicine at UCSF School of Medicine and Founder and Director of the Institute for the Study of Health and Illness. She is author of New York Times best-selling books on medicine, service, and healing.

Rushika Fernandopulle M.D., Co-Founder and Chief Executive Officer of Iora Health, an innovative health care services company based in Cambridge, MA, building a new model of primary care practices nationally. He is Inaugural Executive Director of the Harvard Interfaculty Program for Health Systems Improvement.

Gurpreet Dhaliwal M.D., Professor of Medicine at UCSF. He is an expert in clinical reasoning and was featured in The New York Times as one of the nation's leading diagnosticians.

4) Resident and Student Leaders

Daniel Nagasawa, M.D., Neurosurgery Resident at University of California, Los Angeles Medical Center and former wide receiver for the University of California, Berkeley football team.

Elana Miller, M.D., Psychiatry Resident at University of California, Los Angeles Medical Center.

Renée Betancourt M.D., Chief Resident in the UCSF Family Medicine Residency Program.

Robin Manseur, Student Body President at the Duke University School of Medicine.

Kristy L. Hamilton, Student Body President at the Baylor College of Medicine.

Amol Agarwal, Student Body President at the University of Pennsylvania School of Medicine.

Prologue: The View From The Other Side Of The Bed

What I assumed would be an ordinary day in November of 1997, turned out to be anything but ordinary. Since I was old enough to understand the words "my life has been changed forever," it never occurred to me that one day that idiom would ever apply to me. We move about our daily lives taking everything for granted; our family, our friends, the beauty that encircles the change of seasons, the gracious use of the language, the cutting edge of logic, the wonders and powers of science, or the sounds of rush-hour traffic moving beneath the overpass on Beacon Street in Boston. Clearly there are thousands of people, places, and things that represent the beauty in the world but for some reason, these came to mind on that not-so-ordinary day in November of 1997 and as I walked back to my apartment and, for the first time in my life, I whispered those works to myself, "my life has changed forever."

Receiving a diagnosis that you have a chronic disease is about as far from a positive or pleasant experience one wants to ever have. It's even more distressing when you know that this disorder has no cure. You ask yourself over and over again, "why me?" and thoughts of leaping off that overpass to the Massachusetts Turnpike ran through my mind. What stopped me was the young doctor who gave me the news. He always had a wonderful bedside manner about him and took great care with and of me since my first visit to him five years earlier. There was something about him from the very beginning; I trusted him from the moment we first shook hands. That trust made it easy for me to enter into a wonderful partnership. It's commonly referred to as the patient/doctor relationship but it always felt like so much more than that. Professional but deeply personal at the same time because I shared with him deeply personal and intimate details about my life; things I shared with no one else and through it all, he never judged me. He treated me with dignity, grace, and respect.

I hear his voice in my head frequently even after all these years despite the fact that for the past 12 years, I've been under the care of another extraordinary doctor (I moved from Massachusetts to North Carolina). The Boston doctor urged me to fight. He urged me to live, laugh, and love. Before moving to North Carolina, I met with him one last time. He wept as we hugged and said good-bye. He told me that I was one of his favorite patients and that it has been an honor to care for me. That was the third day in my life (the first was the death of my mom and the second, that day in November of 1997) when I realized that "my life had been changed forever."

While my life has changed in so many ways, what has remained constant is the tender and compassionate care I've received from my doctors. I've always stepped back in amazement at the sheer volume of information doctors have to process in order to perfect their craft and it humbles me. Ironically, my life's journey has brought me to a place where I interact on a daily basis with remarkable young women and men who have chosen to dedicate their lives to human service; a absolute "must-have" for anyone considering medicine as a career path. The science and technology aside, it is the human touch, the softness and tenderness as they speak with me, discussing the good and the bad, the smile and the pat on the back when entering the room, the reassurance that "we" are in this together. All of this has made it possible for me to move forward after all these years. I've also found strength in the shared vulnerability of others. When you recognize that you are not alone, you don't feel like you're alone and it makes the uncertainty of tomorrow bearable.

My doctor in Boston and my doctor who cares for me now are the epitome of "heart." I am reminded every day of the importance of "living" rather than simply "surviving." I'm reminded of the importance of "living rather than simply surviving" during each visit to my doctor. I reminded that the science and technology play a role in my "living" and I have never felt so strongly that the grace, dignity, and respect integrated into my treatment plan have brought me this far.

Every birthday, I celebrate the privilege of growing older. A former medical student reminded me to never lose sight of this. He's right; despite the challenges, the uncertainty, and the occasional obstacles, it is a privilege to be alive and I celebrate every day of my life by laughing with and hugging the extraordinary people in my life, including my doctor.

Richard S. Wallace

Duke University School of Medicine

I have had Crohn's disease for more than 60 years. I was 27 when medication no longer controlled my symptoms and I underwent the first of several major abdominal surgeries. The surgery removed a large part of my intestine and left me with a permanent ileostomy. Unquestionably this surgery saved my life. The only problem with it was that I felt maimed by it. As a single young woman, I felt separated from everything elegant or feminine and from all other women my age. In the week after my surgery I became profoundly depressed and began contemplating suicide. I was a young doctor at the time and hospitalized in my own training hospital. Unwilling to embarrass my colleagues by committing suicide on their watch, I began saving my sleeping pills and my pain pills and making plans to commit suicide when I went home.

In the week I was hospitalized I was visited daily by many professionals, among them enterostomal therapists, a group of young women my own age, who changed my ileostomy as I could not do this for myself. They would come into my room in their white coats, put on a gown, an apron , a mask and gloves, and skillfully remove and replace my appliance. Then they would discard the mask, the apron the gown and the gloves, go to the sink in my room and very carefully wash their hands. This did not help me accept the profound changes in my body. It humiliated me and made me deeply ashamed. But late in the week a young woman I had never met before came to change my appliance for me. She was not wearing a white coat, but was dressed as if she were going to meet a date. Smiling, she approached my bed saying her name and asking my permission to change my appliance.

I was lying there in an outrageous frilly black lace nightgown covered with tiny black bows, a gift from friends who knew how profoundly depressed I was and were trying to be of help. For a moment she just took in all that lace and all those bows. Then with a grin she said "Fabulous! Where did you get it?" It turned out her new boyfriend had a thing about black lace. So we started to giggle together about men and their weakness for black lace and as we were laughing in the most natural way imaginable, she reached into my bedside table, found a new appliance and removed and replaced my old one using her bare hands.

I was stunned. I was after all a young doctor and the first thought that went through my mind was "How unprofessional!" But she continued to talk and laugh with me and I started to watch what she was doing. Her hands were gentle and feminine and her nails were painted a pale pink. No professional woman wore nail polish in those days. She was standing so close to me that I could smell her perfume. No professional woman wore perfume either. I myself did not even wear make-up. And suddenly I felt a rush of strength rise up in me from some deeply hidden source and I knew I was going to be able to DO this thing. It would not be easy but I could make even this radical change in my body all right.

Now this young woman did not give me back my intestine. Medical science cannot do that even today. What she gave me back was my life, not because of her expertise but because of her willingness to touch me with her bare hands and treat me as a fellow human being.

As a patient I discovered that the power we physicians have to heal far exceeds our power to cure. The Healer's Art, the course I developed 23 years ago at UCSF, is now taught by faculty in more than half of American Medical schools and schools in seven countries abroad. The first year I taught it, I asked one of the students what he had learned in the course. "Oh," he said, "I learned that I can heal with my humanity things I can never cure with my science and my expertise." I too have learned this, but at a time when I was wearing a black lace nightgown and not a white coat.

I doubt that this young woman remembers me or knows what the 15 minutes we spent together 49 years ago has meant to me and made possible for me. I do not even know her name. We have all healed many more people than we know. Curing is the work of experts. Healing is the work of fellow human beings.

Rachel Naomi Remen MD

UCSF School of Medicine

Foreword

Health disparities are preventable differences in the burden of disease experienced commonly by individuals worldwide, including those in the United States. They can be explained, in part, by the social determinants of health, such as economic stability, education, social and community structure, and access to healthcare.

You need not look far to identify subpopulations facing health inequity. For example, many Americans have limited access to fresh fruits and vegetables within close proximity of their neighborhoods. In 2011, 83.6 million Americans — 27% of the population, did not have a healthy food retailer within their census district (CDC). They live in food deserts and are more likely to eat cheaper, less healthy foods. While this may be a more economically feasible decision in the short-term, it increases their risk of developing serious chronic conditions, such as diabetes, cardiovascular disease, and obesity.

Access to fresh food is lower among residents of rural, low-income, and predominantly minority communities, which correlates with increased rates of chronic disease in those populations. Although this is just one of example of inequity, it illustrates how disparities impact the health of specific subpopulations and ultimately the health of our patients.

Many of the physician-leaders you will meet through this compilation have devoted part of their life's work to addressing health disparities. Each leader has a unique story and was inspired to take action based on his or her experiences. These actions have many forms and include leading national organizations to advance the interests of patients, directing national health research and policy, and guiding successful medical school training programs to educate the next generation of physicians. In short, these physician-leaders are distinguished individuals with a common desire to serve both their patients and society, making them great role models for aspiring medical students.

While practicing medicine, you will come across health inequities, some which may resonate more strongly than others. There are many ways to respond with the goal of health equity in mind, and each response must be tailored to the challenges it seeks to overcome. You should not feel compelled to act in the way that a physician-leader mentioned in this text may have. Though these physician-leaders have done phenomenal work in their respective fields, I challenge you to resist the temptation of picturing yourself in their shoes. Their actions were often based on their intrinsic motivation to address unacceptable hardships. This motivation, and its accompanying inspiration, tends to evolve organically as we experience the world around us and critically assesses how it affects others.

Given the current landscape of healthcare, we need physician-leaders who are conscious of the social determinants of health and the disparities that are frequently associated with them. With this knowledge base, they can collectively lead the way towards a brighter tomorrow. Each of you has the potential to be a physician-leader, and it is, in part, a conscious decision that you must make for yourself.

I hope you enjoy reading this text and begin to develop an understanding of what makes some of our current physician-leaders tick. I encourage you to explore the breadth of efforts being undertaken to address various health disparities outside of this text, knowing full well that more needs to be done to overcome them. Many patients lack a voice in society, and some of them will be your patients. You are in a unique position to represent them along with thousands of others. So, embark on this quest to learn how health inequity impacts innumerous lives in our world today. And keep an open mind, allowing yourself to be inspired by the people, places, and predicaments around you.

Hussain Lalani

Duke Medical Student and Bill Gates Millennium Scholar

U.S. National Physician-Leaders

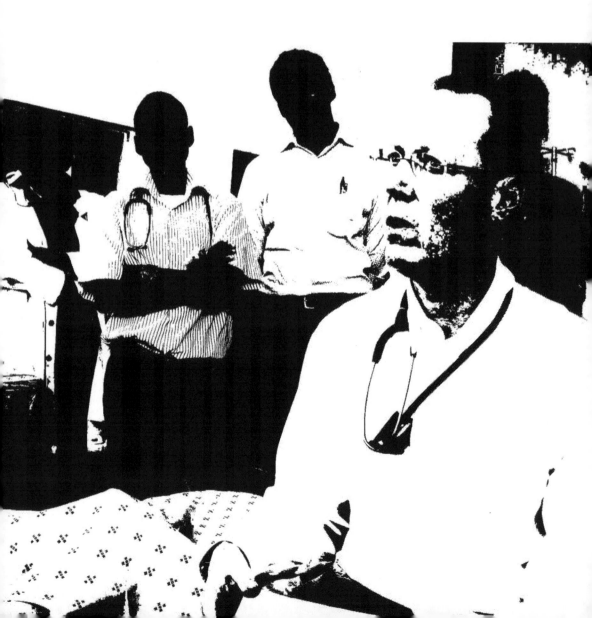

Ardis Hoven

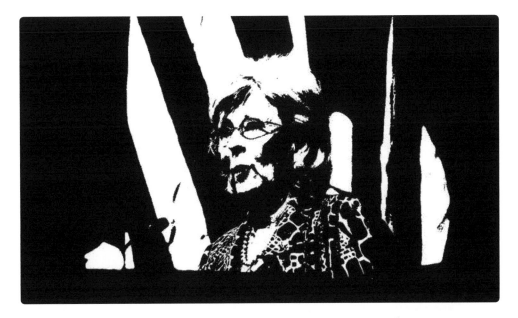

Ardis Hoven M.D. is President of the American Medical Association.

our white coat - This is a great series of questions. It's quite complex. Let me start first with what I perceive the white coat to represent, at least for me in my generation. I think the white coat implies certain things – it implies trust, it implies responsibility, it implies compassion, it implies that I put you, the patient, first. In that sense, the white coat belongs to me as a physician, but it also belongs to patients at the same time, simply because of the elements that our white coat actually represents. Putting on that white coat says I am now going to be the type of doctor, the type of physician, who is going to deliver on what I think this white coat represents.

To the second question, it is important to talk about the fact that the patient is always at the center of care. If the patient is at the center of care, communication is bidirectional, education is bidirectional, I will teach you how to take better care of yourself or I will advise you on the best course of action of a certain problem. At the same time I'm going to learn from you and get feedback from you. But it's always important for me to focus on the patient sitting in the middle of the conversation and look at it from the patient's standpoint. We're both working together, toward better health, because then I can deliver the best possible care to you. But I also want you to be able to freely talk to me about your issues, concerns, your fears, and at the same time we will share in your process of your healing. That's how I look at that whole relationship between patients and doctors.

attending to the world - That's pretty easily stated. As a physician, you are a mentor, a teacher, a role model, a caregiver. By work that you do, you are providing service your entire life. Our entire professional being is centered around serving others. It's not just the patients we serve, it's the health care community, our peers, our colleagues, young men and women we are teaching, our community where we live and work, our responsibilities in our own community to produce tools and wisdom - a variety of things that enable a community to grow and its own health care system. It is particularly important in this day. If look at the way we are changing - trying to change the way we deliver health care in this country. The role of the physician in the community - all health care is local. It's going to be vitally important to making sure we get it done correctly.

uplifting the medically underserved - I wish every physician in this country would wake up in the morning and consider this issue. For me

personally, when I talk about access to a physician, I'm talking about health. Access to health care can include access to clean water, good food, dry shelter. I think they're all interrelated. One cannot have health without having food, water, and shelter. Access to a physician and meaningful health care is just part of that equation. When you go back and look at my career in medicine as a physician, it began early. At the onset of AIDS epidemic here in my community, I was the only physician in private practice who was taking on AIDS patients - we didn't know the cause. There was great fear and great stigma. Many of the HIV doctors throughout the United States were doing the same thing at the same time. In my community, I was no different and my community was no different. What happened was that these patients who had been employed and had health insurance, were losing their health insurance. They got sick and couldn't go to work. They lost their health insurance at a time when they actually needed it the most. For the first time, I saw how the absence of health care insurance impacted the health care system and on care for that individual. The absence of health insurance often led to great fear and great suffering, on top of the fact that they had this disease at a time when they were stigmatized and no one knew what was going on. That propelled me to become a spokesperson in my local state medical association. At that time we were dealing with how this disease would affect physicians and what rules, laws, and policies were needed to protect patients. It was just a stressful time. I became a spokesperson advocating for patients and doing the right thing for the patients. At the end of the day, this is the right thing to do for everybody. This led me to pursue leadership positions at my state medical association and then on to the American Medical Association.

At the AMA, my issue was helping the uninsured access healthcare and continued to be so during my support of the Affordable Care Act. Policy of the AMA, which I helped develop, had to do with helping the uninsured. My role started at home, with leadership and health care access and making sure we were doing the right thing and translating it to a much higher level of function at the American Medical Association. It's been an honor serving as president of the American Medical Association, being able to demonstrate and verbalize healthcare leadership has been important to me.

For me, this all started in the exam room treating patients and keeping that perspective as a leader. You start in the examining room with that patient, or in the operation room or in the ER. It starts with understanding what that patient needs, and why they need it, and if they're not getting it, what's wrong with this system. That's where you start thinking about how you can change the system. It happens one patient at a time. It's that patient - that one patient that makes the light bulb go off in your head and say "listen this isn't right. I need to do something. What can I do?" That's when the challenges start. But as a leader, you can feel gratification from doing something good - when things are not always that way in our country.

a loving smile - Bonding for me says that we were able to share an idea, an interest, an experience or something like that. It's shared. It's a form of communication, I think, and can be done in a very professional way. The best example of bonding was somewhere in the 90s – with many of my AIDS patients. I encouraged them to do this because many were so talented in art –painting, photography, you name it. One of the joys that we shared, not that we had a lot to share because we're taking care of the disease the medications, but what we enjoyed sharing was their artwork. I first started taking care of a young man when he was 6 years old and he started giving me his homework. Another young man was a photographer. He was so fearful from dying. He did a photograph called my daily dose. It was a pill bottle and in the periphery you could see the other pill bottles.

Another young man described it as how his brain felt. For me this is how we kind of shared good things. We talked about their successes. This is difficult but this is what worked for me and it helped the patients too.

a life apart - When and if we lose our ability to feel emotion, to feel sad when something bad happens to a patient - they die, they're bound to have a bad problem - a cancer or a degenerative neuro disease- when we lose our ability to be saddened or concerned, we lose our humanity. And we lose our humanity, we don't need to be doctors any more. That's simply at the core of everyday activities of what we do.

It's in our root. It's in our system. It's in us. Loss and sadness are a part of everyone's lifecycle and we have to be a part of that. When it happens with the patient or the patients family, you have to be able to accommodate it you can't let it run you over. Somewhere early on, I learned how to do this or maybe I was taught by a mentor. When I walk into an exam room with a patient or a patient's family, that is the only thing I am going to think about. I let all the other noise fall away.

When I'm with a patient, yet I've just lost patient, I can compartmentalize my sadness and direct my energy on to the new patient and a new problem. At the end of the day, I know I have given the best I could possibly give, all of my energy. At the end of the day I gave them the best I had, and if I know that, I can move on to see the next patient. You have to compartmentalize, but that does not mean that you lose the humanity, you lose the compassion, or all the pieces I've talked about it, but it gives you time to heal a bit and move on and take care of the next one and the next one. I saw that during the AIDS epidemic. As I walked down the hallway in my hospital here. At one time I had patients in every private room on one floor of the hospital. One was sicker than the next. I would go from one room to the next room. How do you function? How do you keep yourself improving and what you're going to do the next patient. When you're in that room with that one patient and that one patient's family or friend, you give them everything you've got. Then you move on and you go to the next one and you do the same thing. You bring to each patient, you bring the highest energy, the highest level of compassion, and you'll do the right thing.

a story - I'm going to tell you two stories. This occurred when VRE was just emerging in our ICUs. Our young mother had been given a medication, developed severe pancreatitis, isolated for weeks and weeks, had to get surgery, and long story short, she developed a VRE bacteremia. At that time, one of partners was going off to a meeting. We were all involved in taking care of this young woman. We got to know her family, her children. Each day we hoped and prayed that you had an answer to the next problem that would arise. My partner came back from meeting – she said, let me tell you about this new drug, it's an experimental drug. We've got to get it for our patient.

By golly, we started rolling things around at the hospital. We got the IR people to agree to it. They let us use this new drug which became linezolid. It was so exiting. Everyone in our intensive care team, the nurses, the pharmacy team, the laboratory folks. Everybody was so excited about this and it was probably going to make a difference and in fact it did. It saved her life. I get Christmas cards to this day. She's adopted another child. She's healthy and doing great. She has a family.

What's inspiring is that it took one person going to a meeting, that went to another meeting and then said let's try this. Not being passive, being aggressive. We got everybody involved in it. It was one of the celebratory things when we saw it working and her recovery after months and months in the hospital, going home. That's the kind of thing that makes all the long hours worth it, that's the kind of thing that makes working together worth it. How important that team care piece is for what we talk about in healthcare today.

Story 2 has to do with a young man with HIV/AIDS that his mother died of. He came to me when he was 6 indirectly, because I had cared for his mother. She presented with CNS lymphoma and she died shortly after presenting. I didn't know there was a child involved. I looked at the chart and I said this is a child, I don't do pediatrics. The nurse said "you're going to do this one". The boy came and was HIV infected. He was 6 years old at that time, he wasn't ill. I continued to take care of him up until now. He's alive and doing well, He was never hospitalized. We managed to slug our way through various medicine combinations. Along the way, as he grew older, here's a young man – good looking young man- having conversations about protection.

He said, 'Doc, if you wanna talk to me one more time about the birds and the bees, I'm walking out of here.' Today he's a healthy young man, 28 or 29 – I forgot how old he is, doing well. That's a wonderful story. That can happen. The role you play for someone along a continuum is extremely important as well. This goes to the relationship with a patient. This guy was 6 and he was brought in by his grandmother after his mother had died. He was being cared for by aunts and uncles. His mother was mentally disabled, she was raped and that's how she acquired HIV. This little boy was old enough to remember his mom and grew up knowing what happened. The importance of his family, his grandmother, his aunts and uncles, and the community supporting him. Part of that community was my office and the need for the healthcare team in my office to be involved. I think it's a very important lesson.

The VRE story goes to collaboration and team care. At the time it was happening I wouldn't have called it that. It was before the time we focused really focused on team care. This was truly team care.

a lens into your life - When I became president-elect to the AMA, I went into a part-time position simply because I knew I would not have the ability to try and see patients and consistently be there when they needed me and do my work at the AMA. I made it clear that my job at the AMA was my real job for the next three years. The challenges of my work as the leader of the AMA are significant but they are also very rewarding. My job takes on various shapes and forms, a communicator to the health care community at large, communicator with members of Congress and those in Administration at the national level. As we walk through the Affordable Care Act implementation, and as we're looking now in other changes to the Affordable Care Act, as we're addressing issues around Medicare payment and reform, as we are addressing issues around delivery changes that need to take place to this country, and also movement in the quality arena, all of which I have been active in the last few years.

My job is phone calls, communications, meetings, document reviews, looking at what we can communicate, how we need to do it and how we effect change. A recent example was spending about two days at Capitol Hill, meeting with our staff at the AMA, meeting one on one with leaders of Congress who will be working very diligently on payment reform and payment and issues. Speaking with members of Congress on their staff, educating them, hearing what they have to say, answering their questions, giving them information. That's a large part of what I do. I do that with media and with my colleagues here at home. I'm writing a letter to my own local medical society. It goes to the fact that I am the person responsible for making sure that the message of the American Medical Association is delivered appropriately. I love talking about our three focus areas. I love talking about the fact that we are looking at medical education in a way that has never been looked in the United States before and how we're going to accelerate change in medical education. I love talking about our improved outcomes activities – around getting patients with hypertension blood pressure controlled, preventing type II diabetes. I'm very much involved in groups of folks around this. Thirdly, one that I'm passionate about is practice stability, sustainability and sufficient satisfaction in healthcare delivery. All of these activities are ongoing and evolving and I am very much involved at a high level at making sure that every-

one knows what we're doing, how were doing it and are we working in the right direction.

That's kind of the core of my job responsibilities over the last three years. The other thing that I do is the three presidents (current, past and future) of the American Medical Association are the three representatives from the United States to the World Medical Association. As a consequence of that I've had my eyes open globally around health care and access to care. It put a new, better understanding of how not only we need to deal with things at home, but how we translate what we know in the world. I'm in the learning curve of that. These are exciting times. An ideal day for me is having every member of the press love what I say and print it just exactly the way I said it and everyone reads it. That would be a perfect day for me.

I'm very passionate about health care. I'm very passionate about patients and patients being at the center of things. I can remember AMA working to pass the Affordable Care Act and I've said this multiple times since then: if it's not good for my patient, it's not good for me as a physician, and it's not good for the health care community. If you look at that space between the patient - the space between the patient and the doctor is a very sacred space - a sacred space that we as physicians need to protect. And that's my job.

Darrell Kirch

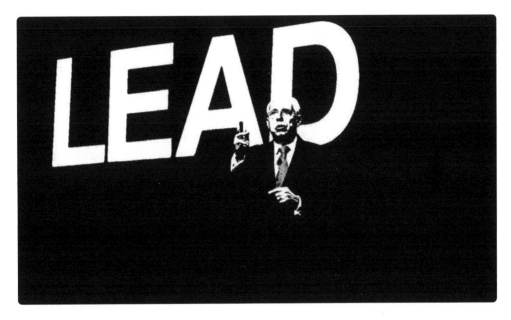

Darrell G. Kirch M.D. is President of the Association of American Medical Colleges

our white coat - When I speak at white coat ceremonies for medical schools, I am always struck by how unnatural the coat appears to feel when first donned by students. When they receive their coat at that ceremony, it is simply a stiff, starched garment. In the years to come, the white coat will become increasingly meaningful to each physician only through the encounters they share with each other and their patients. The white coat is simply a piece of fabric, and its true meaning is derived from the experiences of the individual wearing it in relation to the experiences of the patients they seek to help.

attending to the world - I do not consider this to be just a personal opinion, because I believe physicians' dedication to public service is prescribed by clinical ethics. Almost any textbook on clinical ethics emphasizes core principles, not only beneficence, doing no harm, and respecting the patient's autonomy, but also virtually every explication of clinical ethics includes a commitment to social justice. My conclusion is that it is impossible to be an ethical physician and believe your responsibility extends only to the patient in front of you. That patient must be put in the context of the community and society. Serving society is an inherent ethical obligation. This is not an option for physicians. It is an ethical commitment, not an elective.

uplifting the medically underserved - Defining access to a physician as a human right is simply too narrow. The human right is to have access not only to a doctor, but also to wellness and health promotion. To preserve health, it is of utmost importance to engage with a number of health providers beyond physicians. Certainly, universal access to a physician would be an inherent social good, but the basic human right to health is more than simply the services of a physician. For those of us who have the privilege to work with and lead national organizations, one of our greatest challenges is the presence of health disparities and inequities. In the United States, we are one of the world's richest nations, yet our current system has created "haves and have-nots" when it comes to health care and to the ability to experience a healthy life. These inequities should be a source of national shame and should motivate all of us, regardless of our chosen health profession, to confront and correct this injustice.

a loving smile - For physicians directly involved in patient care, bonds are important in building trust with patients. The ability to simply smile

and demonstrate a sense of humanism can be very valuable tools in establishing this human bond. The bonds forged with patients should be in each patient's best interest, and there are boundaries that should not be crossed because they can harm the patient. For example, engaging too much in revealing your own personal information or intruding inappropriately into the patient's life can impair the trust a patient feels. Patients do not want cynical, emotionless physicians, but they do need to have a core sense of trust. One of the key competencies for a physician is to know where the boundaries are and to not cross them. The best clinicians I know consistently show explicit emotion and empathy, but never cross the line of familiarity in an inappropriate fashion.

a life apart - To be devoid of emotion, especially the capacity to feel saddened in the face of suffering, would severely limit a physician's ability not only to give care, but to be caring. At the same time, it is important to not allow oneself to be overwhelmed by these feelings, but to find the ability to transform emotion into productive energy to serve each patient who is suffering. I think it is important to show emotion, especially empathy, in front of patients, but more importantly, to show emotion in front of medical students and resident physicians. Trainees learn through each attending physician's actions. If those actions demonstrate to a trainee that a physician needs to build up an emotional armor that is impervious to the plight of the patient they are seeing, that is a tremendous disservice to the patient and to the learner. At the same time, learners and physicians alike must not cross the line of letting our emotions interfere with our best medical judgment, our decision making capacity, and our capacity to do the right thing for the patient.

a story - Even though I didn't choose to pursue obstetrics, I always have felt that one of the most meaningful things we are privileged to do as physicians is to be present at the birth of a child. It is the most extraordinary, intimate moment of life. It is an incredible honor that, in your process of becoming a physician as a medical student, you are allowed to share in that joy. It is an event that very few are allowed to share. I always find myself telling medical students, especially early in medical school, that this will be the kind of experience that will help them realize the special privilege they have in being part of our profession.

a lens into your life - For me, it is not just a single day, but a repeated experience. When I was an actively practicing psychiatrist, some of the most despondent people, with perhaps the greatest suffering I have ever observed, were patients with severe depression. They simply could not see any light at the end of the tunnel, which is why, sadly, some commit suicide. Encountering a patient who is severely depressed and giving them a sense of hope and saying with confidence that I believe they could get much better, possibly in just a matter of weeks, if they would work with me on their treatment plan is an incredible privilege. To help someone, who may have been experiencing true misery in their life, reach this turning point defined for me the "art of medicine." Those experiences also allowed me personally to find meaning in medicine by, in turn, bringing hope and meaning into other people's lives. Even in the case of a dying patient, we, as physicians, can give the patient hope that they will have a "safe passage" through the end of life. My best days are those where I have the privilege of instilling hope—whether that is for an individual patient, the next generation of physicians, or in our society.

Deane Marchbein

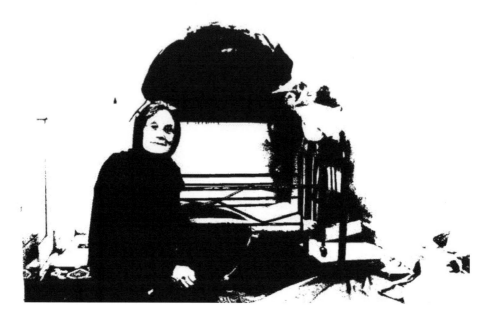

Deane Marchbein M.D. is President of Doctors Without Borders.

our white coat - This is an interesting metaphor because when I am in the field I do not wear a white coat. The white coat is a way of establishing authority and hierarchy and not really what I believe in. There is understanding that I serve people in the developing world in states of crisis or when a natural disaster takes place. What I wouldn't want to do is put up any sort of barriers, because my effectiveness depends on a meaningful cultural exchange that helps people to make choices, using my expertise and respecting their beliefs. The sort of interesting thing is that I realize you are choosing the white coat metaphorically. I think it is a problematic metaphor for physicians.

attending to the world - I look at the physician as a care giver, as somebody who has a core body of knowledge to share and skills to share. I put that the center of my life service to people who would otherwise not have access to care. I help the people who are around me, I don't know if I believe in attending to the world. I choose to be in places where the people deeply need someone to be there for them.

uplifting the medically underserved - I would dispute this idea. It concentrates on one person doing something to the other. There is really a disparity in the role of societal physicians. Contrary to the idea of physicians offering service, access to medical care I definitely believe is a human right. Without access to healthcare and good health, it is really impossible for a people to be successful. Whenever it is a question of fairness, I think that we should all have access to decent healthcare.

a life apart - When I stop feeling and having a connection with the people I serve, when I stop feeling sad about the condition that I see, it is time for me to think about doing something else. The empathy that we feel, whether as physicians with patients, or as physicians with trainees is important. I think that engagement and connection is core to the therapeutic relationship, and core to our humanity. I do see a lot of things that are plain outrageous and sad. I talk to colleagues and tell myself in most cases that I didn't cause this mess. I am just there to do what I can; I can't be responsible for everything that I see around me. I will not always succeed. At the end of the day it is about helping and doing no harm. Sometimes you don't succeed ; that is just the territory.

a loving smile - Not sure I know the answer to that question. I feel a deep bond with my pa-tients but I'm not sure that they reciprocate. That is not something that you can expect. Someone once said, proverb, that if you help someone you own them. We set up an OR in an area in the middle of a war zone. It was this aid, the presence of an OR and a surgical team, that saved a woman's life in front of my own eyes. I sometimes wonder if they forget about me or their experience in our hospital. But I'm not sure that's such a bad thing that they are able to go on with their lives and forget. Moreover, I am always amazed when I see children overseas and they don't cry when something hurts. When you give them a shot, they have every right in the world to cry and be difficult. I feel very sad that often these children have so much suffering that it doesn't occur to them to act out in any way. They live out the experience and move on. I learn a lot from them as a physician and I also learn a lot from them as a person and patient myself.

a story - There is one that I take with me every time I go to the field. So I was in the Congo, where any woman worth her salt delivers a home with no help. They wouldn't reach out until they were in pretty bad shape. There was a woman who had walked for several days straight, and she was pregnant and in labor, and her uterus ruptured. The baby was dead and the only question was whether we would be able to save the mother. she was bleeding, and the surgeons struggled to gain control. The mother had a cardiac arrest, and the mere idea of doing CPR was the most ridiculous thing imaginable. When someone arrested, it was pretty much game over. We didn't have a blood bank, we didn't have a ventilator, we didn't have anything that a modern hospital would have. I thought of her seven living children without a mother. the idea brought me to tears. I thought,'Not on my watch'. I didn't have a proper anesthesia machine, but I just jumped on her chest and started doing CPR as someone else squeezing blood in. At the end of the procedure she managed to wake up. We had no intensive care unit. The nurses worked the overnight shifts for 18 hours. Those working at night often had other jobs during the day. We kept her in the recovery room and kept up these shifts for a week and a half. They kept her alive. they transformed our little recovery room into an intensive care unit just for her. Finally, we were able to move her back to the ward. The next week, we all started going to the market and buying extra special healthy things for her to eat. Then basically the woman left the hospital. It wasn't what I did; it was getting to share in something wonderful that I will always remember. It was a time of war in Congo. There were almost no resources, let alone money to buy her food. Our lives alone were in immense danger. Yet, everyone chipped in together and went to the market together, we became a team to make this woman and her family survived. May this be a vivid demonstration of the awesome power of empathy, of being willing to be there for anyone.

a lens into your life - There is no average day in my practice, and that is what is so interesting. Sometimes I am giving direct patient care and providing anesthesia at Harvard Medical School's affiliated hospitals and clinics; sometimes I am teaching local nurse anesthetists and nurses how to give anesthesia in times of need; sometimes I am setting up anesthesia equipment and operating rooms in places where there has never been one in history. Sometimes I am the global physician who prepares people to successfully deliver intensive care in moments of crisis. The excitement and the interest in my work for me is that it is never the same. And I get to serve constantly. I love what I do. I really do. But this isn't mutually exclusive, come join me.

Francis Collins

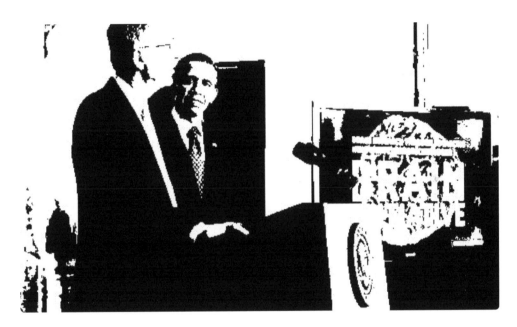

Francis S. Collins M.D. Ph.D. is the Director of the National Institutes of Health.

our white coat - My main job is serving as the Director of the National Institutes of Health (NIH), overseeing biomedical research for the United States. Those heavy responsibilities don't allow me time to see patients, except occasionally as part of a research project. But the things that I learned wearing the white coat as a medical student, as a resident, and as a practicing internist all instruct and influence me every day.

Here's one example: any decision about how to invest in medical research that lacks patient engagement is impoverished as a result. The voices of patients, more than ever, are perhaps the most critical ones to consider as decisions are made about priorities. I spend a lot of my time listening to patients and disease advocates, wishing that NIH had more resources because we can't pursue all of the scientific opportunities that are available. But if NIH research is going to have any success, it will be because we are linked tightly and meaningfully with patients, whom I consider to be our partners and co-investigators.

a story - Let me share a story from my first experience of trying to deliver care in the developing world. The setting was a small rural hospital in a very impoverished part of Nigeria. When I arrived there for my two weeks of volunteer service, I thought that my Western medical training and my attending physician experience at the University of Michigan would prepare me for everything. But I quickly discovered that most of the problems I encountered were way outside of my reach. Not only were many of the medical conditions that I saw unfamiliar, but I also came face-to-face with the stark consequences of poor or non-existent public health services: lack of clean water, lack of vaccinations, and lack of access to care.

After a few days, I got quite discouraged and began to question why I was there. Somehow, a 26-year-old Nigerian farmer that I was treating for tuberculosis sensed that. When I came to his bedside on rounds, he surprised me by saying, "I sense that you are wondering why you came here." It troubled me that my self-doubts were that obvious. But this patient had an answer: "I'll tell you why. You came here for one reason: you came here for me." And suddenly, it all made sense.

As much as we as physicians like to imagine ourselves as large scale healers of the world, when it really comes down to it, what counts is the one-on-one interaction with someone who needs your help. So, if you ever find yourself feeling inadequate, remind yourself that every healing effort matters, every relationship with a patient matters, that's what it's all about.

attending to the world - Other peoples around the world have far fewer resources than the United States, and that continues to be a significant motivator for me. One of my highest priorities at NIH is global health research, to see if we can implement some of the scientific advances happening here in ways that will help those that are not so fortunate. Of course, this mandate not only applies to helping people in other lands, but to helping the less fortunate within our own borders.

I also place a very high personal priority on addressing health disparities. All of us in medicine should feel disturbed when we look at the evidence that different groups are experiencing very different health outcomes and opportunities for care. At NIH, we fund research to identify the causes of such disparities, and then we develop and test interventions that will improve these discrepancies. Of course, NIH is part of a very large ecosystem of research and medical practice, but I think we can play an important role in providing the evidence needed to change unacceptable situations in which economics, race, and ethnicity are affecting peoples' chances of living full and healthy lives.

uplifting the medically underserved - Access to health care should not be a privilege, it should be a right. At NIH, we are doing everything we can to support that right by using our research to identify ways that make it easier for all people to have access to health care.

However, I would challenge the assumption that access to healthcare has to equate to access to a physician. In some parts of the world, where there are so few physicians and so many in need, there are ways in which alternative approaches using health care extenders can be enormously useful. That's what we're doing now with programs like PEPFAR in countries that have a high incidence of HIV/AIDS. Many of those countries do not have significant numbers of physicians to deliver antiretrovirals , but other healthcare extenders are doing that quite well.

Personally, I see reaching out to the medically underserved as one of the strongest drivers for what I do. I would not be comfortable presiding over an enterprise that felt otherwise about the importance of healthcare for all people. The Bill and Melinda Gates Foundation, with which NIH works quite closely, has as its motto that every life has equal value. I agree. And that means that part of my responsibility in setting research priorities is the preservation of each life, and doing everything possible to encourage that life to be healthy and flourishing .

a life apart - When it comes to interacting with patients and mentoring trainees, I think physicians who refuse to show any sign of emotion reduce the practice of medicine to something more mechanical and less humane. To give a recent example, my laboratory works on a rare disease called progeria, which is a form of premature aging. This is a disease that affects only about 300 kids in the world, but it is heartbreaking to see what happens to them as their bodies age at a rate about seven times faster than normal. Over the past 10 years, my lab has devoted a lot of effort to research on this disease. We found the genetic cause, and the next step was to come up with ideas about therapy, and then see those therapies enter a clinical trial, which showed benefit in terms of slowing down the cardiovascular disease that normally takes the lives of these children about age 12. But it is not a complete success story.

One of these wonderful kids, Sam Berns, died in January of this year at the age of 17. I've known Sam and his parents since he was 3 years old, interacting with them on efforts supported by NIH and the nonprofit group they founded, the Progeria Research Foundation. Upon hearing the sad news of Sam's death, I changed my schedule around at NIH and took the day to go to Boston to be part of his funeral. I wanted to grieve with lots of other people whose life has been touched by this very wise and brilliant young man. For the sake of Sam and all of the other patients whom we have loved and lost, I think it's inappropriate to pretend that their deaths don't affect us. In fact, I think it is good for a physician to show some emotion in front of the medical team and trainees in such situations; otherwise you are depriving them and yourself of the opportunity to be fully involved.

a loving smile - There has always been a tension between the relationship that one naturally feels as you get to know another human whose health you are trying to assist with, and the need to remain objective about delivering bad news and making medical decisions. I confess that I've probably tipped in the direction of being pretty comfortable in more transparent relationships with patients; I just can't imagine how you can enter this intimate place in someone's life when they are facing some really serious medical challenge, and fail to do it in a fashion that involves your entire being and not just your medical knowledge. I can tell you that it results in a bond between patient and physician that offers both parties the potential for increased meaning, as well as increased vulnerability. Still, I don't see how you can practice medicine any other way—a cold, robotic style wouldn't't work for me as a patient, and it doesn't work for me as a physician.

a lens into your life - My life at NIH provides me with a marvelous opportunity to be able to survey the entire realm of medical research; almost every day there is something that comes across that landscape that is breathtaking. Just today, we were all marveling at two papers in the journal Nature that show that you might be able to make pluripotent stem cells from mice (and maybe people too) simply by taking white blood cells and putting them under stress with low pH. That is just completely unexpected, totally astounding, and carries all kinds of potential consequences, in terms of what it might mean for future cell-based therapy for lots of diseases.

A really great day for me is when my team gets to announce an ambitious program that creates new and unprecedented scientific opportunities. For example, on April 2, 2013, I stood next to President Barack Obama as we announced a pioneering effort to understand how the human brain works—how the circuits of the brain do all the things they do in terms of complex deliberations, making decisions, laying down memories, and retrieving and processing information. We need to find out what goes wrong in those circuits at a very fundamental level if we are ever to treat and prevent conditions like autism, schizophrenia, epilepsy, traumatic brain injury, and Alzheimer's. Yes, that was an excellent day. It doesn't get much better than launching a project like this that electrifies the scientific community, holds tremendous promise for medicine, and has the strong support of our nation's leaders, even the President of the United States himself.

Image: Dr. Collins introducing the BRAIN Initiative with President Obama. Official White House Photograph. Contributed by Dr. Collins. Credit: Chief White House Photographer, Pete Souza.

Harvey Fineberg

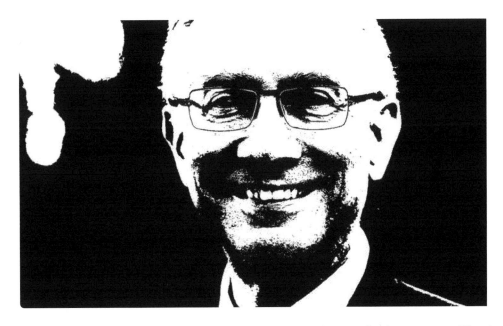

Harvey Fineberg M.D., Ph.D. is President of the Institute of Medicine, Provost Emeritus of Harvard University, and Dean Emeritus of the Harvard School of Public Health and Partners Healthcare.

our white coat - The idea that the patient is an equal partner in care is now a well-established principle, but we have to think beyond the individual's immediate medical needs. Our responsibility is caring not just for the whole patient, but caring for the whole person as well. That means understanding their life, and their circumstances at home and in the community. When it comes to physician decision-making, being a partner sometimes means also being willing to take responsibility when patients want you to direct their care in the way you think is right. You have to take responsibility for your role in their life and responsibility to understand their needs at each stage of their illness. The key idea I would say is to treat the patient as a whole person. Additionally, it is important to understand your role at that moment in time, for that particular individual in front of you. Being a physician calls for different ways of interacting at different times. I think that the idea of patient-centered care is truly about care that incorporates the beliefs and preferences of the patient.

attending to the world - I have not been an attending physician for more than twenty years. I have mostly been in an administrative role. When I did care for patients, it was a very special responsibility, one that all students, trainees and attending physicians share. It is a position of trust, it is a position of great personal content, it is a very special opportunity to serve and do something worthwhile.

uplifting the medically underserved - I have always believed that health is a fundamental right. If you look at the constitution of the World Health Organization, it declares that the highest attainable standard of a nation is a fundamental right of every human being. In the U.S. constitution, there is no specific guarantee of a right to health. About 86 countries similarly do not have such a constitutional guarantee. Notably, many countries without a constitutional guarantee nonetheless have programs and commitments to honor a right to health for all of their people. A desire for equity leads naturally to a belief in everyone's right to health. Without such a constitutional guarantee in the United States, it is nonetheless possible, by our own collective choice, to honor a right to health. We still have an important challenge ahead of us.

a loving smile - The most important tools are your two ears. Listening is the most important tool. Always.

a life apart - I don't think you can be a good physician without compassion. You have to have a sense of deep awareness, and identification of the needs of your patient. There is also a kind of compassion from a certain distance, which is necessary to protect yourself. Sometimes we confuse professionalism with a lack of emotion. You can be professional and still show patients that you really do care. I don't think it is always unprofessional to show emotion, I think it is human. I think it is a natural part of living your life in medicine, while remembering you have to protect yourself from emotional burnout.

a story - I don't know if I have a single story that would inspire a first year medical student. Everyone has a story about what it is that made them want to become a doctor. In your whole career it is important to return to that story. It is important to remind yourself what made you want to be a doctor in the first place. I still would come back to the idea that as long as you treat every person in front of you as a whole human being, not a collection of symptoms, not a list of medications, not a pattern of diseases, but rather as a whole human being, you'll make a positive difference in your career.

Joanne Liu

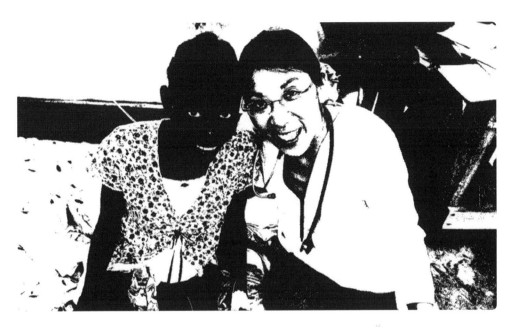

Joanne Liu M.D. is International President of Médecins Sans Frontières (MSF), the umbrella organization of Doctors Without Borders.

our white coat - The white coat belongs to the symbol of medicine. In low income country where health care access is scarce, the vision of the white coat for some might be hope of care. Saying all this, since I am a ER pediatrician, I never work a white coat but scrubs in ER. I was told very early on that white coat frightened children.

attending to the world - I have never questioned the basic premise to serve patients of all backgrounds. Being Canadian where we have social medicine, it is a given. I decided to become a pediatrician and I wanted the world to be my emergency room. I remember distinctly in Darfur in 2004 when I worked as a pediatrician in the nutritional centers. There were hundreds of patients in our waiting room and each day, we had to send back patients home without being seen. People arrived in poor conditions at the beginning of the emergency and initially, we could only attend to the critically ill patients. Often, the world just doesn't fit MSF emergency room.

uplifting the medically underserved - Again, from my perspective, access to health care is a must and we should strive for a world where everybody has this access. We should cherish it where it exists and we should fight for it where it does not exist.

a life apart - I think that sadness is a normal human emotion in times of loss. I often work in contexts where one cannot take the time to feel sorry for oneself, but in due times, one should take the time to process those emotions and share them.

a loving smile - In MSF work contexts, our most precious reward of our work is the smile from our patients; to see a malnourished child running up the feeding center after few weeks on treatment recovering her ability to smile is priceless.

a story - When I work in war torn zones with Médecins Sans Frontières(MSF), I am always amazed by the combativeness of my patients and their attendants. Sometimes, mothers have walked weeks to come to a MSF clinic, braving checkpoints, intimidation by armed rebellion or looting, to say the least with a sick child on her back. In response to their incredible resilience, I always find it a hard match as a care taker but I am inspired by them.

a lens into your life -I think that every day is my best day. I have the most fulfilling job either at field level when I work as a pediatrician or when I deal with governmental authorities of a given country for access to an underserved population.

Kristen DeStigter

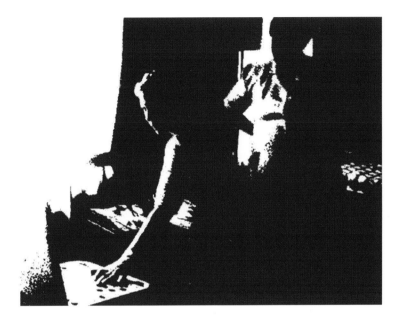

Kristen DeStigter M.D. is John P. and Kathryn H. Tampas Green and Gold Professor and Vice Chair of Radiology at the University of Vermont College of Medicine. Dr. DeStigter is Founder of *Imaging the World*.

our white coat - My name is Kristen DeStigter. I am a Professor of Radiology at the University of Vermont, College of Medicine. I am Vice Chair of the Department of Radiology at Fletcher Allen Health Care in Burlington, Vermont. In my role, I manage all operations of the Department of Radiology including quality assurance, pa-

tient safety, and clinical work flow. In addition, I am the residency program director wherein I mentor and help train 24 Radiology residents.

As a passion, I co-founded the non-profit organization, Imaging the World, [www.imagingtheworld.org]. Our mission is to bring the highest-quality, accessible and affordable ultrasound to rural health centers in sub-Saharan Africa. Currently, we operate in Uganda. Our program trains midwives at the point of care to perform antenatal ultrasound examinations for pregnant women.

Imaging the World began with a basic premise: Too many women and their unborn children are dying from complications associated with pregnancy and childbirth that are preventable – complications that can be easily diagnosed by ultrasound. ITW's ultrasound and teleradiology solution is integrated at the point of care in rural health clinics. It is accompanied by a sustainable train-the-trainer program, capacity strengthening of human and system resources, community education, a robust patient safety and quality assurance program, and a sensible business model, all geared towards saving countless lives.

attending to the world - When I chose to become a physician, I dedicated myself to a life of service to humankind. I came from a family and parents who were completely devoted to helping other people in need, and I was the first person in my family to ever become a doctor. Why I chose this socially responsible calling as opposed to others, I do not know.

As a physician, my purpose in life encompasses many roles that all seem to gel together. When I travel to Africa, I am accompanied by high school, college and medical students, medical residents, and other physicians, nurses and technologists. I use these trips as an educational experience to extend my work and service in Africa and to encourage other people to do the same.

uplifting the medically underserved - I believe that every person has the right to high-quality, safe, effective and appropriate medical care. As a Radiologist, an educator, and an expert in global health, my role is to bring highly accurate, reliable, and affordable diagnostic imaging services to the most vulnerable people in rural locations.

a loving smile - I believe in bringing the patient into the medical decision-making process. One way to do this is to educate and inform the patient about what is going on inside his or her body. This is something physicians can do with ultrasound at the point-of-care. In rural Africa, ultrasound results are discussed with pregnant patients and their families, allowing them to know in advance of the time of delivery if there is a potential complication and to plan for next steps. Then, they have the time to prepare for the journey to a hospital where they can get a C-section, if needed. By bringing the patient into the decision- making process, we are saving lives.

a life apart - Our emotions identify us as human beings, and one cannot be a good and effective doctor unless those emotions exist and can be outwardly expressed. Being able to speak to a trainee or converse with a colleague or talk to a patient and show emotion is not only a gift, but a necessity in the practice of medicine.

a story - There was very young pregnant woman in rural Uganda. Like all of the women she knew, she decided to give birth in the village with a traditional birth attendant rather than go to the health clinic. But there was a problem in childbirth – she labored for four days at home and was near death when her family finally brought her on a motorbike to the clinic. An ultrasound scan showed that she had (unexpected) twins and that they were both presenting foot-first causing obstructed labor. With this knowledge, the midwife was able to turn the presenting fetus so that it came out head first. This allowed both babies to be delivered successfully and the mother and her two children survived and are living in the village today. This was the first "save" in Uganda because of Imaging the World. We call these events miracles, and there have been so many more since this first time.

a lens into your life - As a Radiologist, I am dedicated to bringing the highest-quality, accessible, affordable ultrasound and teleradiology services to rural, antenatal health centers in Uganda, other parts of sub-Saharan Africa and the rest of the world. As a physician, I am dedicated to improving and saving lives.

Molly Cooke

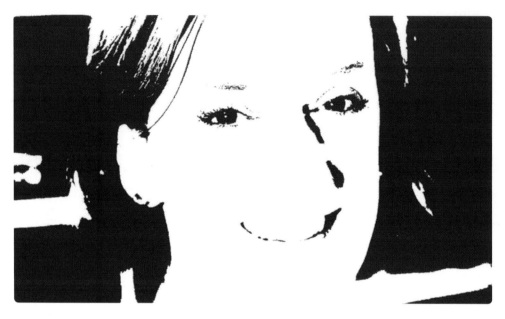

Molly Cooke M.D. is President of the American College of Physicians and Inaugural Director of Eduction in Global Health Sciences at UCSF.

our white coat - I am a general internist, and I do primarily outpatient medicine. The best I can do is encourage patients to address their own health problems, but the patient is going to do 95% of the work. I often tell the residents, if you have a diabetic patient who is on a twice-daily insulin or oral hypoglycemia regimen, that person is going to make 180 choices on how and when to take these medications between every

visit with you, not to say anything about the 3-5 choices every day on whether to eat and exercise. If the patient is not engaged in the prevention of health problems or in the treatment of diseases he or she may have, in outpatient internal medicine we're absolutely dead in the water. Absolutely the patient and physician are in partnership to promote health and minimize the impact of disease.

attending to the world - It's all about serving other people and finding a way to be helpful. Some clinicians get frustrated in settings where, for one reason or other, patients can't or won't do everything that the physician directs them to. To me, that's the wrong model. The model is, how can I be helpful here? That really starts with the patient's agenda. Having said that, sometimes the patient has the wrong agenda. That's where the relationship gets to be very important, because what the physician needs to do in that situation, in my opinion, is work with the patient over time to interest him in at least the most critical features of the physician's agenda. This can be a long, slow process. It's a process of using the relationship with the patient to help him shift from where he is right now to being one step healthier. For a patient who uses needles and doesn't want to stop using injection drugs- and clearly that's my goal for that patient- if they're sharing needles then using a needle exchange program is safer. Is there a way we can work together to have the patient do this in a safer, healthier way? It's a lot of trying to shift the patient's agenda. A lot of times these folks have been berated by physicians and other healthcare professionals. If that's been their experience, it can often take quite a while to build up a real sense of relationship and trust and really convince the patient that what I want to work with are outcomes that the patient values.

uplifting the medically underserved - Health care is a human right. Health care is a big, complicated endeavor. Lots of people play important roles. Physicians are a part of it. A lot of people should have access to physician-informed care, but many people live in parts of the world where they're not going to get the majority of their healthcare delivered one-on-one by physicians. There just aren't enough physicians. We need to get smarter for physicians to interact with nurses, nurse practitioners, community health workers, family members, and patients themselves out of the face-to-face visit. I think all of us have a responsibility to use our skills in training that are the result of a very significant societal investment in us. Everything I know how to do, it's because I've had huge investments made in me by my family, and also by my teachers and the taxpayers. So I'm really a steward of these assets that belong to society. We all have a responsibility to recognize how much has been invested in us and how great needs are in terms of health in our own communities and globally. How can I be most useful in the world?

a loving smile - I've had a discrete revelation about this: I don't have to fit in a box that is physician. I can be a physician out of my own personality and values. I can be more myself than I've previously allowed myself to be. I think that it's always important to at least offer a real person-to-person relationship to each patient. Not every patient wants that. Some people just want their blood pressure medications refilled, and that's fine too. But it really ought to be a patient's choice how much of a connected human relationship they want to have. Having said that, real person-to-person relationships are complicated, and allowing patients to form relationships with me does not mean to me that I don't have any privacy or that the patient is allowed to do anything that he or she wants to do by virtue of being a patient. Recently, a patient was relentlessly critical of everything we were doing in the practice. We were really extending ourselves, but she could only find fault. I said, "Part of a good relationship is to see things from another point of view. Let's think about whether this is really fair to people who are working hard on your behalf." I'm a general internist, so I see patients for years and decades. For this kind of continuous care, some people really value that kind of connection. My youngest child is 26, and I have patients who remember before I got married- they've known me for more than half my life. It goes both ways.

a life apart - If our relationships with people are real, then sometimes we're happy and sometimes we're annoyed and sometimes we're sad. I think that at least for me, it wouldn't be healthy not to allow myself that full range of emotional responses to what I see. I may be less annoyed and sometimes less sad because of the way I frame my work. If I can help patients be one step healthier, I get all excited about that. If my goal is to fix everything, I can hardly ever fix everything, so I would spend a lot of time frustrated. So I just found a way to participate in some of these questions - whether in health policy or poverty in a patient of mine, and how that individual's poverty affects their health without feeling I'm responsible for fixing it all and that I've failed if I don't. There's this big work, and we've all contributed a piece of it.

Paul Farmer

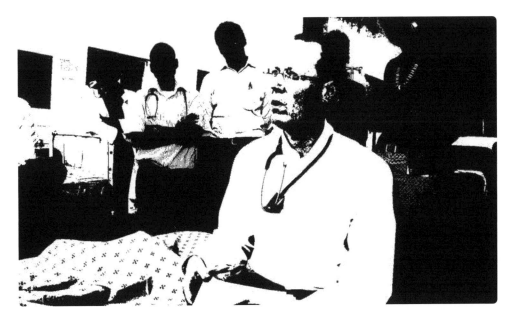

Paul Farmer M.D., Ph.D. is Co-Founder of Partners in health, Kolokotrones University Professor at Harvard University, and Chief of the Division of Global Health Equity at Brigham and Woman's Hospital in Boston, Massachusetts.

our white coat - We were confusing the practitioners with the system. But most of the physicians who I know are deeply committed to the best goals of medicine. We just have a crazy system in the United States - and many places in the rest of the world - that's really not focused on reduction of suffering and protections from unnecessary suffering and disease. They're focused instead on finance and cost-recovery or the wrong incentives for doing a surgical or diagnostic procedure. So that's what the white coat means to me - it's the marker of a certain commitment. I see it certainly in every day clinical practice but also in the medical students I meet at Harvard - a lot of idealism and remember our obligations as healers.

For patients, as healers, I think it took me a while to learn this. In the early part of my medical career and medical training, 25 years ago, I could look back and say that I understood that early because a lot of our patients with tuberculosis were recruited to become community health workers. So that's a pretty literal acknowledgment of the patients as healers. But I think that as time goes by, I keep learning more about this - about the potential of patients to really direct their own care. This is especially true of primary care and chronic disease. This term that rankled me when I heard it misused - "empowered" - I think I do understand the good parts of empowerment as well. How can we allow people to be agents or have agency in their own illness, in their family's illness, and in preventing illness? I think I have a lot to learn about patients as healers, but I've been learning my whole life about it and have a deep interest in it.

[Matt: Do you think that the improvements being made to our current health system are more of a bandaid in terms of getting to a form of pure agency? Or do you think that we should completely eliminate our system and have a system much like Europe?]

I think that what's happening now is that the American delivery system is expensive and nowhere near as effective as it could be. It makes it harder for many practitioners to do their job instead of making it easier. It makes it harder than it needs to be. I don't have ideology feelings about this matter. For example, you mentioned the European healthcare systems - and there's great variation inside Europe and inside one country, a sociological complex country such as France as compared to Norway.

A lot of these European democracies with solid healthcare systems also share a mania for border control. So when you talk about human rights, it's not the same as citizens' rights. It's a right that every human should have. So if we're going to talk about ideology, I'm more committed to the notion of healthcare as a human right rather than the right of a certain system. I know that's not a very common view - and it's probably not helpful for people trying to run national, state or county healthcare systems to have someone come in and talk about healthcare as a human right, but I feel that way. I think that the system that's constituted now offers disincentives for some of these strivings in medicine.

Now I work in Boston at the Brigham at what's probably the best hospital I've ever seen. If you need a heart transplant or if you walk in front of a car and need orthopedic surgery, it's a really good place to go. The surgeons and nurses - everybody - I love working with them, and they have fantastic skills and really great values along the lines of what we're discussing. But that doesn't mean that that beautiful hospital - a research hospital in an academic medical center - that doesn't mean its embedded in a good system. So that's a distinction. I would never discourage any of my undergraduates from going into medicine, saying, "The American system is so messed up, it's just not worth it." I would never say that because I've loved being a doctor in the United States. In regards to improving that system or altering it profoundly, I'll regard that as our shared obligation. I hope that other clinicians and nurses feel the same way.

[Matt: I wish you ran the system and the way that healthcare works, Dr. Farmer.]

It would overwhelm me! I have some friends like Don Berwick who have struggled with this mightily, among others. It's such a complex system that it's beyond my skill. I'm an infectious disease doctor – and the role of each of us in our respective specialties will be in systems improvement. Don't think for a minute that you're not going to enjoy this work enormously in spite of the profound inefficiencies of our system. It's great work – but we could make it a lot easier with these systems innovations.

[Matt: If you want to change the system, would you say that primary care is the way to go? In surgery, there seems to be a lack of direct policy or opportunity to propagate policy towards health equity.]

It's not so much that there's a great deal of opportunity in internal medicine either. Most of the internists that I am lucky enough to work with in the United States, including primary care internists, don't really have much engagement on the systems level. It would be better to have more of us who are involved in this. If you want to be a surgeon, by all means do that. If you want ongoing contact with patients with chronic disease, by all means do that. Finding a way for all of us to get involved, however modestly, in systems improvement and in thinking through some of the policy questions is something that all of us can be involved in. I wish I were more involved in and knowledgeable about the American healthcare system. I'm committed even at my age to learning more and doing more regarding the country were I was trained and teach, which is the United States.

attending to the world - "Attending physician" is by definition a leadership role. In the system here in Boston, it means working with trainees and students and patients and families. Almost all of the care that attendings here deliver is in concert with others. The picture I sent is one of the attending in Malawi, and it always means working with a team, with nurses, with trainees, in the inpatient setting. I think that's a great chance for all of us to interrogate what we might jokingly call our QPE – our quest for personal efficacy. All of us wish to be effective. A hand surgeon who is going from residency to fellowship will be called to be personally effective.

uplifting the medically underserved - I wrote a book together with Father Gustavo Gutierrez called In the Company of the Poor regarding strategies for social justice in medicine, particularly for the poor or otherwise marginalized. He says, "Paul Farmer talks a lot about health and human rights. That's all well and good, but in fact the poor do not have the right to have this right." There are so many barriers for people living in poverty and with critical illness that it remains aspirational in any healthcare delivery system that thinks of services as commodities.

Does that mean that I would say, "Don't be a surgeon because you won't get paid unless you bill for procedures?" Of course I wouldn't say that. I work with surgeons in the United States who find their practice deeply satisfying. The system is set up to disincentivize providing the highest quality of care to the patient. It undermines our ability to have a meaningful discussion about healthcare as a human right.

This is something that I could not have laid out clearly when I was in medical school. I would have said, "Health is a human right. How is that different from 'healthcare is a human right'." I wouldn't have been able to make that distinction very well at the time. It took a long time for me to realize that I do believe in health as a human right, but it urgent we push for an expression of healthcare as a human right. Once someone is sick or otherwise marginalized then the medical profession has to take a stand on providing those individuals with access to care.

For a lot of my friends who are subspecialize surgeons, some of the other experiences they get of not commodifying procedures is in some of the places we work, such as in Haiti. After the earthquake, for example, people came from all over the world to help us. We needed complete surgical teams - anesthesiologists, surgeons, surgical nurses - because a lot of the big trauma was crush injuries, etc. Imagine if we're trying to say, "All right, here's the care you need. We can provide it. And here's the fee." That's essentially what we often do in the United States. It's just that most of the

surgeons I know are not involved in things like billing - and they don't want to do that, it's not why they became surgeons. But that's how the system mostly works, although there will be changes to it, as you all know. Generally, we don't have the infrastructure in a place like Haiti - well, we do now in central Haiti, meaning the new hospital - but by and large, you don't have the infrastructure. This is an opportunity where your subspecialist surgical colleagues can feel good about saying, "Hey, I'm doing this because I think the patient - because they're sick - deserves it."

Surgery in general is less context specific - that's why anesthesia dosing in a procedure are usually not different in one context versus another. So if you have a decent system, you can go in for a relatively brief period of time and make a difference with surgery. This is very difficult to do in psychiatry, general medicine, pediatrics, etc. A subspecialist ICU nurse once she or he has been in an ICU, it's not that different to be in a different location. In primary care nursing, however, the context can make quite a difference. So, when you have a surgeon who goes back to the same place, and fitting into the same system that he or she has helped to build, focused on local capacity building, I think that is a very legitimate model. So I don't discourage short-term medical missions if they fit in that kind of model. Unfortunately, a lot of them don't - often it's a group of providers who have a week, bring in their own meds, and they're not part of an essential drug list or a pharmacy system, and they're trying to deliver primary care, and it's nowhere near as sound as trying to invest that passion into developing a local delivery system. Getting that improved is going to take some time.

a life apart - I wouldn't get too caught up with term "appropriate." I'm going to be in a distinct subgroup of medicine because I hear the use of that term all the time. It is a sociological construct - what is appropriate gets redefined over time, it differs from place to place. I'll share my views on it. As medical students, as residents and as attendings, you will actually need to decode what is considered appropriate by your team in your context. You have to do it because you're being part of a team. There is a code of comportment that you have to figure out how to decipher. That can be a very good process if it leads to real teamwork. That said, if you're in a field where there is a lot of suffering and much of it unnecessary or premature, then why on earth would it be inappropriate to feel? If the answer is because it prevents you from doing your work, then it requires training and support from other members of the team. If you're a pediatric oncologist, and a 12-year-old kids dies in front of you, which is devastating to a family - this happens all over the world, although it happens less in the United States - I don't think it's appropriate not to think of it as appropriate to be deeply saddened by such loss.

When you're an attending, I think it's very important to promote compassion and empathy. I'm not advising you to chat about this all the time - you have to be aware of the code of comportment of a busy medical team. Whether you're an internist or a surgeon, just as with any small group of people, you have to know how the team works and keep the focus on the patient. I wouldn't be too confident that there is an easy answer to this question beyond the fact that of course it is appropriate to feel sad and of course it is appropriate to share your sadness with your teammates - and also with patients and their family members.

Now, how is that best for the patient? That is the critical question. In my own experience, when someone gets bad news as a patient from me, I work very hard to be optimistic and cheerful and encouraging. And I think that's what a great majority of patients want, in my experience as an infectious disease doctor. There are exceptions to that. There was a patient of mine who almost died in December, 15 years after being saved from tuberculosis and AIDS following proper therapy - and he almost died from tetanus! I was sad and almost terrified by that. Fortunately, he recovered. I also felt some shame and disappointment as well. I would encourage you to have non-disruptive ways of expressing these emotions - especially to the patient, but also to the team since their focus is the clinical care of the patient. Most of the hospitals are now trying to do a better job, walking away from overdue confidence that one sentiment is less appropriate than another. The question is, is it disturbing to the patient or the family members or is it disruptive? Often you'll find, in my experience, that it's not - that actual, families in pain appreciate knowing that their physician and nurses are sharing that with empathy and compassion. That's from my experience as a clinician.

a loving smile - Of course a loving smile is welcome in the clinical setting. I don't think it matters at all, what your area is. A loving smile from a hand surgeon is just as welcome as a loving smile from a primary care physician. I have serious doubts about the notion of the term "appropriate" as you can tell. You can say, "context appropriate" or "situationally appropriate" – the trouble again lies with disrupting the team. In most clinical care, you don't want to disrupt or derail or disturb. We are, as physicians, in the business of "caregiving." You might look at the writings of my mentor, Arthur Kleinman, for examples of this. I'll tell you one story about him. His wife, who was a very good friend of mine, had early-onset dementia. She had a very painful, slow decline over the better part of a decade. Arthur Kleinman, who is a physician-anthropologist, became her primary caregiver, and this involved many interactions with the healthcare system. He learned a lot about how there isn't much focus on caregiving even with a chronic illness like that. Some of the best parts of the difficult years were loving smiles and emotional support from professional caregivers to his wife - but also to him, and to the rest of his family. I do think medical students, residents and fellows are almost obligated to understand codes of compartment in order to be effective members of a team - it's not about you

and your quest for personal efficacy, it's about high-quality care for patients.

I keep thinking about you guys rounding with your teams. What's hard for an intern often is understanding that code of comportment. The rest of the team doesn't want you "practicing your loving smiles" during busy rounds, right? But there are lots of ways for even a surgical resident to have contact with patients and their families – even in a busy teaching hospital. I would encourage it. The interns are the ones with the craziest hours, but I've had a very positive experience, and I know that our trainees have too. We have a new surgical intern in Haiti, and I went to see a patient – a young woman, a school teacher, who we thought had leprosy and had neuropathy in her feet, in any case. She had come in with a serious infection that I thought for sure would require amputation. So far – as far as I know – she did not lose her foot, and that was thanks to the surgical team who debrided her wound – they were just consulting me about antibiotics and what might be done. What struck me was that she said to me – and remember this is a schoolteacher probably living in poverty, probably who only makes a couple hundred dollars a month – she said, "The doctor was so nice to me, he was so pleasant." And I said, "Which doctor?" And she said, "Willy." And I said, "Oh, the intern!" So I went back to the intern and his attending, who is a very experience, well-known Haitian surgeon, and I said, "Let me tell you what this patient said. She said, 'I really like how compassionate he was.'" And that wasn't during rounds, showing off – that was him going back and sitting with her. Imagine being 30-something years old and having leprosy that's made you almost lose your foot. How are you going to get around in a place where you can't get a prosthesis? I was very proud of him, and I wanted the rest of his team to know that that's never going to go out of style or become inappropriate to be kind and concerned and worried and have a loving smile.

Your peers in med school and in training – they are people in their twenties. You've never been sick or seriously ill. I got hit by a car as a medical student, and I still wasn't really "sick." I couldn't walk for six months, but I never really felt "sick." And I certainly didn't think I was going to die or be disabled. As Americans, you probably haven't lost any siblings, your parents probably didn't die when they were in their twenties or weren't disabled by things. So allow yourselves as trainees to acknowledge that it's the same set of emotions that people feel in the rest of their lives. The real challenge, though, is not to enable your feelings of self-interest or self-pity or self-indulgence – that's not good. What is good is sadness for others or grief, when appropriate, for others' families – a loving smile for others. A loving smile that you gives yourself in the mirror, that I'm not for. [Laughs.] But all of these – ambivalence, anxiety – why not? You're talking about serious matters, and that's true in internal medicine too, not just trauma surgery or pediatric oncology. It's true in every field in medicine, including radiology or pathology where you're not necessarily even with the patient. But the patients are still patients – your patients. Sometimes there's nothing you can do but just think, "What a shame. This is so sad." There's nothing they can do, but you can at least acknowledge that fellow feeling for someone in unfortunate circumstances.

In closing though, most of the emotions are joyful. It is pleasure and privilege to practice medicine. If you've got the right delivery system, then it's a pleasure and privilege to deliver surgical care, for example, in the middle of central Haiti. It should be, but you've got to have the tools of the trade and the team that's required to deliver good care.

Another thing to think about when you're taking about service-minded physicians is that no service is beneath you. Do not think that because you're an attending or a doctor that there are "nursing duties" that you don't do – that's ridiculous – or other kinds of pedestrian, unglamorous tasks. It's not about what you consider glamorous or the opposite of pedestrian – it's about what's need to deliver good, effective, and compassionate care.

a story - I couldn't come up with a favorite story – I'll make one up shortly. I've had so many experiences that have been instructive to me, from everywhere that I've practiced medicine – Boston, Haiti, Rwanda, Russia, etc. I've had such a varied kind of practice, that I have lots of them. Every year, I try to write some down for one purpose or another. I just was thumbing through this book of speeches, and I pulled out a story that I used for a graduation speech for an undergraduate school. I had to think about some of the hard lessons I learned in my twenties. Even though they are hard lessons and painful, that doesn't mean they're not inspiring. There are all kinds of ways to be inspired. If you think about some heroic advance – lets say the discovery of a new antibiotic that's going to change people's lives or the first kidney transplants – those are really important stories to know. I think right now, one of the things I'm most excited about is the story of how science and clinical needs, including the science of trials, is resulting in a new curative therapy for chronic hepatitis B. That's not a personal story in the sense that I had any role in it, but it's inspiring to me. Think about the possibility for people who have not been curable. Most of the ones I know are people living in poverty or marginalized because they're in prison or have another illness that we've been involved in addressing - for example, drug resistant tuberculosis or HIV disease. Now I think, wow, how terrific is it that over the course of only a few years we've gone from seeing a chronic and often lethal infection transformed into a curable disease?

The story that I thought of in sharing with you is really about delivery systems. It's really about, "Do we have an equity plan for hepatitis B medications?" Not that I've heard. It should be, "Your access to this wonderful new set of therapies is going to be based on your clinical need and not on where you live or what kind of insurance you have, etc." That's a narrative that I learned in many ways the hard way when I was

in Haiti and was your age. I had this experience that I still think about, being out in the village and being involved in a community health meeting after walking a long way. This was after I had gotten hit by the car, so I had already had the experience of receiving good medical care so that I was able to walk miles and miles and miles again. I was very, very lucky because I had been hit by a car in Cambridge, Massachussetts as opposed to rural Haiti. Even if I had been hit by a car in rural Haiti, I probably would have been air-lifted out of there. Anyway, having only one medicine in my pocket – an inhaler because I asthma. I didn't have a diagnosis of asthma as a child – I actually got it as a Harvard medical student. This lady came up to me and said, "Please come see my husband. He's really sick. He can't breathe." My first response was, "I don't have anything on me. I don't have a stethoscope, I don't have medicine. There's nothing I can do here – bring him to the hospital." I say "the hospital," but it was probably still more of a clinic back then. She insisted, and I wasn't gracious and finally acceded. I was walking in the wrong direction now, and my leg hurt a little bit. And when I saw her husband, I knew it was status asthmaticus – this young man was dying of asthma. And the good part of the story is, of course, that he lived because that was the one medicine I had in my pocket. So speaking of delivery systems, it's hard to get that medicine into him because he couldn't breathe at all. So that was scary. But the delivery system he needed was community-based care for chronic disease. So these kind of experiences taught me a lot about the role of health workers, transport, making sure that care was available to and convenient for the patient, not for the providers or the providers-in-training.

This story inspired me first by dread because I thought, "That was almost a colossal mistake on my part because he would not have survived getting to the hospital – or not likely." It was inspiring at first, but later in reflecting upon it over the next twenty years, I've worked on building better delivery systems and safety nets in that part of Haiti.

I've worked with a lot of people, and the secret to the service-minded physician's success is always going to be teamwork. The team was there, in this case – the community health worker asked me to talk to this lady. It was my inattention to what the community health worker was saying. I didn't tell this story to have me be inspiring. On the contrary, I wanted to share with you how uninspiring we can be or almost be, and how we need others to pull us out of that. We can make errors – that story was almost a disaster – but when you are part of a team and can work with other people, you can really make a big difference.

a lens into your life - January 31, 2013, Neno, Malawi, examining a patient at Neno District Hospital with local clinicians, visiting Global Health Equity residents and Harvard Medical School students. Photo credit: Rebecca E. Rollins / Partners In Health.

Sir Richard Thompson

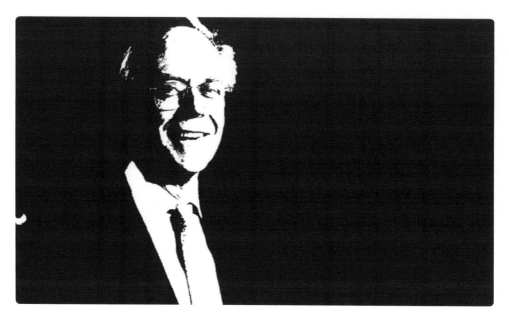

Sir Richard Thompson D.M. is President of the Royal College of Physicians in London.

our white coat - The doctor is a healer but the patient takes part in healing themselves, and the physician leads and advises.

attending to the world - I think the attending physician does serve other people and thus we call it the National Health Service in the UK. Part of a professional physician's remit is to do the best for the patient in front of them, and you can certainly call that service.

uplifting the medically underserved - I certainly believe it is a human right for the poor and the ill and the people who are suffering during wartime. They should all have access to a physician, and it's worrisome that in some parts of the world it's not the right of a physician to attend to people who are rioting against the government.

a life apart - I don't think it's appropriate for a physician to be sad in front of patients or trainees, but they can be serious. They should not show emotion, but they can certainly demonstrate that they have empathy. Potentially the physician should be cheerful at all times, which is important for patients in their recovery. Even if patients are very ill, they are very happy to joke with their physician. It's important to encourage humor throughout medical practice.

a loving smile - If patients want the same doctor looking at them, it's the right thing for a patient to be with the same doctor all the time, good for them and for their relationship. Then the patient gets to know the doctor and knows that the doctor is following their illness. I think it's important if it's possible, thought it's not always possible.

Thomas Frieden

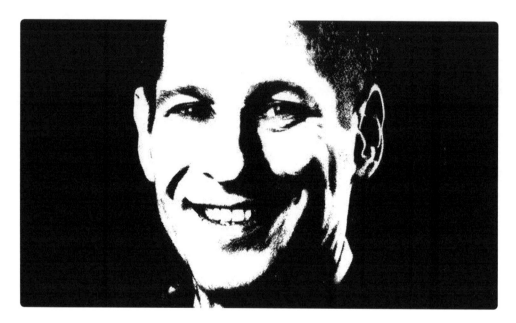

Thomas Frieden M.D. is Director of the U.S. Centers for Disease Control and Prevention.

our white coat - One of our top priorities at CDC is to strengthen collaboration between the health care and public health communities. This is perhaps crucial over the next decade. Health care and public health are like two wings of a bird - both are needed to fly. Health care providers focus on the health of individual patients, while public health is concerned with the health of entire communities. On a fundamental level, we try to help individuals reach their full potential, and the work we do in public health to improve health at the community level supports that goal. If you look at the past 100 years or so, the greatest health improvements have come from public health initiatives, such as clean water and air, strengthened tobacco control, improved industrial and environmental safety, cardiovascular disease prevention, and many others. Our health care system needs to pay better attention to patients - and our public health system can help them do that by being an "honest broker" of information, bringing public health knowledge into clinical care. We highlight the most important health problems facing our country, implement the most effective ways for both the health profession and individuals to address these problems, and foster ongoing discussions to achieve these goals.

attending to the world - New technologies make our world smaller every day. But increased globalization brings increased risks – the threats we face are greater and so is the ability of microbes and disease to move more quickly and farther than before. A disease outbreak anywhere is a threat everywhere, and the next pandemic may be just a plane trip away. CDC works 24/7 to protect the American people from threats, whether infectious or non-infectious, naturally occurring or man-made, originating here at home or in any part of the globe. At CDC, we strive to maximize medicine's impact and our own activities are part of the greater national effort to help people live the longest and healthiest lives possible, both here at home and throughout the world. What is exciting about public health is that we make meaningful contributions not just to one patient at a time, but to whole communities and even entire countries. That is why I hope every doctor considers entering public health. With passion, we really can change the world and improve the health of millions of people.

uplifting the medically underserved - Equal access to health care and preventive services is a fundamental aspect of human rights. As Martin Luther King said: "Of all the forms of inequality, injustice in health care is the most shocking and inhumane." Everyone should have an equal opportunity to live the longest and healthiest life possible, and advances in both public health and medical care can help us achieve our goal of health equity. CDC identifies and addresses factors that lead to health disparities among different racial, ethnic, geographic, socioeconomic, and other groups so that barriers to health equity can be removed. There are many ways we can make a huge difference through work with populations in greatest need. We need to address disparities with solutions that can be scaled up to cover whole communities and the entire country, as well as solutions that address specific problems such as diabetes, in ways that best serve those who are in greatest need. As a physician, you should want to be part of a medical community that addresses disparities and anything else that might impede the best treatment for each patient. It is the most ethical and fulfilling way to practice.

a life apart - Two things that I've found to be important as a physician are the ability to actively listen, and a sense of humility. As a doctor, you need to listen to your patients to make an accurate diagnosis. And you have to listen to what they're not saying as well – sometimes, what people don't say is more important than what they do say. Physicians also can't possibly know everything about everything all the time. Knowing that you have to be aware that there is always something you don't know is incredibly important – it can make the difference between life and death. So is trying to extend your knowledge, not just for your research work and career, but also for each individual patient's health and safety. In my career, I've learned an enormous amount from nurses and pharmacists, who very often have a better sense of what a patient needs. Nurses are working more consistently at the point of care, and pharmacists have specialized knowledge about medication issues that many physicians do not. Too often, I see young physicians who downplay the expertise of other health care professionals, and this is a big mistake. It is important to recognize the expertise of all members of the health care team, and that everyone working together and drawing on each other's knowledge is in the best interest of the patient. The more you personally learn as a physician, the more effective you can be. The more you understand patients and their specific situations, the more appropriately you can and will respond. Knowing yourself better will also help you become a better doctor.

a caring smile - It is critical that doctors develop effective communication with their patients and relate to them as individual human beings and not merely as one in a series of patients. The lives of our patients are at their core much like our own. If we lose this perspective, we lose the chance to make perhaps the greatest impact that anyone can make in any career. I love clinical care - it's why I became a doctor in the first place. Looking back at clinical experiences, I enjoy having the chance to make the same type of impact for whole communities.

a story - A pivotal moment for me came when I was put in charge of tuberculosis control in New York City in the midst of what by 1990 had exploded into a raging TB epidemic. This was my first assignment after my time as a CDC Epidemic Intelligence Service Officer – a "disease detective" – and I was determined to do everything I could to reverse the epidemic. We hired staff, improved clinics, expanded outreach, educated doctors, and went to the bedside of the most difficult patients. A few months later, Dr. Karel Styblo, one of the world's pre-eminent tuberculosis experts and one of my personal heroes, came to town. We were proud of our hard work, and eagerly showed him detailed diagnosis and treatment data on each patient. But then Dr. Styblo, after reviewing detailed statistics on the program that we had published, asked me one question that changed my life – "How many of these patients did you cure?" I had no clue, and was terribly ashamed. I had to go back to remember the essence of accountability to each patient, which led me to hold myself and the program to a much higher standard. We then went back to make sure that every level of the program was accountable for results. And we succeeded in stopping the epidemic, and to this day the program successfully cures nearly all of New York City's TB patients. We all have to answer Dr. Styblo's question – "How many people did you cure?" – in whatever form applies to our work to maintain the accountability we owe to each patient, and you must ensure that every other person on your care team is doing the same thing. It is critical that we meet each challenge in medicine with complete care and perfection, and with rigor, to best serve patients.

a lens into your life - There is nothing more satisfying than helping cure someone from a serious health condition, whether tuberculosis or heart disease, or a serious risk factor such as tobacco addiction, which continues to be our leading preventable cause of death. Helping to cure individuals from something that causes enormous suffering and affects their ability to live a long, healthy, and productive life is something that you never forget. In public health, we can save not just one person, but thousands or even millions. It is incredibly exciting. One thing we strive to do in public health today is to help people see the faces and the lives behind the numbers.

team-based medicine - Our clinical care and public health landscapes continue to change rapidly. Ultimately, we need to make sure that physicians are fully integrated into health care teams and accept support from other team members. It is inevitable, as our health care system becomes more efficient, that we will make use of every member of the clinical care team to have the maximum possible impact. We need to provide care that has protocols in place to ensure that each member of the team listens carefully to what each patient says as well as to their other team members. Nurses and pharmacists as well as lay outreach workers are all crucial members of our country's medical teams. Technical expertise is essential, yet insufficient. Please never forget that. It is critically important to develop both technical and interpersonal communication skills as a means of effectively supporting a team and helping patients. But sometimes in medical school, there is a divide. Each of us needs technical rigor as well as the capacity to listen to patients and work well with others. We are a discipline that, first and foremost, is and needs to be about people.

Health System and Medical School Leaders

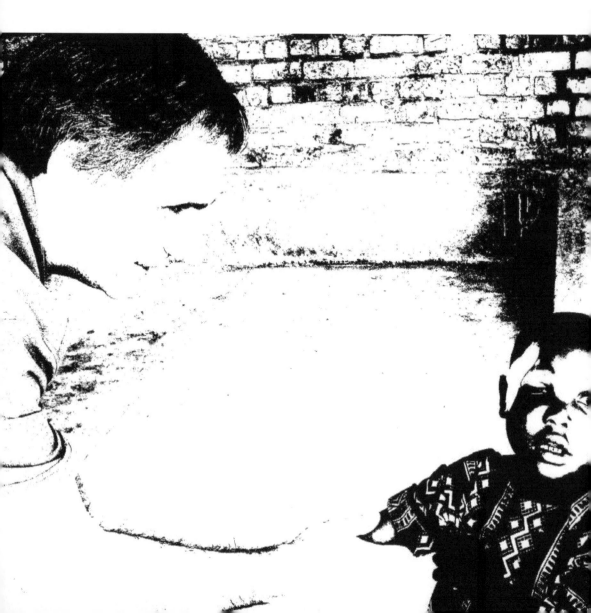

Anthony Atala

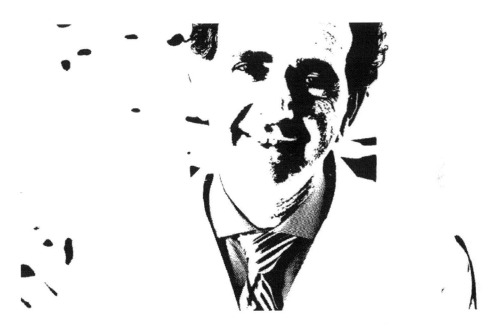

Anthony Atala M.D. is W.H. Boyce Professor and Director of the Wake Forest Institute for Regenerative Medicine, and Chair of the Department of Urology at the Wake Forest School of Medicine in North Carolina. Dr. Atala developed the first lab-grown organ to be implanted into a human.

our white coat - I'm a pediatric specialist. Often I go without wearing a white coat when I'm with my patients in the pediatric population. I try to bring something in the room that's child-friendly. When I'm walking in the hospital hall-

way, I have a white coat on, which helps to identify me as someone with access to the patient room. But if it were up to me, I wouldn't wear the white coat. I want to encounter the patient on a human-to-human level, and the white coat can sometimes get in the way of that.

Even though I'm in a pediatric surgical specialty, my job allows me to have patients for many years. I have patients who I operated on when they were born, and now they're college graduates. Having the ability to see patients long-term is not about the white coat, it's about the personal relationship you have with that patient and family. To me the white coat is not a reflection of medicine in general. It's actually something you have to get beyond to be able to get to know the patient in a real way.

attending to the world - That's what motivated me personally to become a physician. The path may seem long but it's really brief. You have a choice early on in in life: Are you going to enter a service-oriented profession? For me it was a no-brainer; I wanted to provide a lifetime of service. My life took many different turns on my path toward being a physician. I became a physician but also a researcher. It was a path of, how can you always provide service to others?

That really has been a major driver for me. How can I be of service to others? That applies when I'm seeing a patient one-on-one, seeing a family, teaching medical students and residents, and even in my research career. It has led me to understand that by treating patients one at a time you're helping that one patient; by then taking that knowledge and using it for research, you have the potential to not just help one patient at a time but many patients at the same time.

uplifting the medically underserved - Health care is a right. As a society we have to be able to get together and make sure that the right basic needs of service are provided for everyone. Health is one of them. Obviously people are responsible for their own health. At the end of the day they have to live responsibly. There's education that goes behind that, and it's so important.

But also if something does not go right, then you have to provide that health service for that patient. There *is* no other option. There *should* be no other option. There *must* be no other option.

We are in a world that has always felt that providing health care is a very important piece of our humanity. If you look at war conflict, what happens? People go to the battlefield; they fight each other and try to injure each other. But in the armed services hospital, they take in all injured: they take injured from their side, they take injured from the other side. If you go into the military unit in Afghanistan or Iraq or in one of the other conflict areas, you'll see patients who, just a few hours before, were fighting each other. When they walk through those doors, they're patients. They're human beings, and we take care of them.

So the concept of human health is not just reserved for the few or the favored; it's available to everyone. It's critical that we as a society work hard not just to make sure everyone has the right health care, but also the right education regarding health.

a life apart - At the end of the day it's really a human-to-human interaction. You're basically dealing with patients, you're dealing with their illnesses, and you're dealing with their ups and downs. You rejoice with your patients when things go well. You're happy, and you let the family know you're happy. I'm thankful that things have gone well. I'm thankful to the family that they have placed their child in my trust, and

I'm also happy for the child who has done well. It's the same thing if a child presents with a condition that does not have a good prognosis. The family is going to be sad, and I have to recognize the fact that the family is going to be sad.

There's nothing more powerful than sharing your empathy with your patients and families because as humans we have emotions. We have to make sure that families know that you do feel for them and that the emotion that you feel is a direct relation to the fact that you care for them. That empathy piece is very important to the daily practice that you have. I think all the time of patients who have had devastating injuries. I feel for them. I don't feel for them at just that moment, I feel for them for years to come. It's part of who we are as physicians.

a loving smile - You start having a bond with a patient from the very initial contact. When you go through the grocery line, you have a relationship with the person who's checking your groceries out if you go to the same store and go through the same line. If you go to a tax accountant, you build a bond and relationship with her. We are building bonds with people we encounter all the time in our daily lives. It is no different for a physician in terms of establishing that rapport and bond, but it is even more important for a physician to do so.

Just the fact that the family to coming to see you about their child's medical problem implies a certain trust before they even walk through the door. One of the most amazing things to me is that someone can come to me in my office, they've never met me before, and basically a week later I have a scalpel in my hand, making an incision in their child. That requires an enormous amount of trust. It's a trust that is precious. Not only does that trust have to be preserved, but it also can never be violated.

Basically you have to encounter the family and patient on a personal level, a one-to-one level. You have to let them know you're really watching out for their best interest. Your actions and words have to be accurate and reflect that you do care for them. Not only will you care for their health problem, but you in fact do care for them as individuals also.

a story - I was walking past the Intensive Care Unit as a medical student. The nurse told me that a patient, a lady in her 60s, was not doing well. I approached the patient with my stethoscope and listened. I thought, Oh my gosh, it sounds like this patient has a cardiac tamponade. This is a condition where the heart is not working as well within its cavity. So I called the resident who said, "Get the blood levels." The patient was declining fast, so I called the resident back. I said, I really think this patient will need surgery to have this taken care of. They said to me, call the cardiothoracic surgeon. I called the cardiothoracic surgeon, and the patient started to decline fast. I rushed the patient to the OR. The cardiothoracic surgeon was there and said, "Scrub in. I'm going to need your help" because it was so emergent.

We were not even scrubbed when the patient flatlined. Then I watched as the surgeon took a scalpel and cracked her chest open. He had his hands inside her chest pumping the chest. We had not done a total scrub. We had broken all protocol, but he was trying to save her life. He pumped and pumped, and he was very aggressively pumping away. It went on for minutes. To me it seemed like ages. In my mind, I kept saying, We have to stop. We have to stop. She flatlined. Even if she comes back she may be brain dead. Wouldn't you know it? Her heart started beating again. We irrigated that chest cavity with copious amounts of fluid. She was sutured and went back to the unit. Two weeks later that lady walked out of the hospital. That was one of the biggest lessons I had in my life as a physician. I realized that we do not decide when the patients' chances are futile. It is not up to the physician to give up. We should try our very best no matter who the patient is and what the situation is. We should do our best every time.

Charles Sorenson

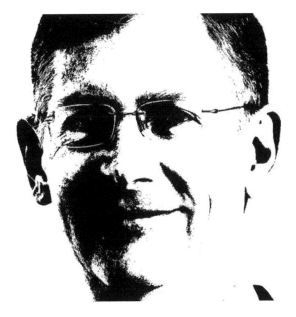

Charles Sorenson M.D. is President and CEO of Intermountain Healthcare.

our white coat - I'm probably a bit old school, so I think ultimately the white coat belongs to the doctor. Of course it's important that both doctor and patient work together and share the healing experience. Still, for me, the white coat symbolizes a lifelong dedication to learning about people, about the diagnosis, management and prevention of the diseases that affect them and how to make a meaningful human connection with others. Using our expertise at the highest possible level and establishing relationships of mutual trust and accountability are important aspects of our professional responsibility. These are the reasons people come to us. The white coat should symbolize our acceptance of that responsibility.

That said, you won't find anyone who is a greater advocate for stronger participation by patients in the choices that affect their health. We, as Americans, often don't think it's our problem when we make unhealthy lifestyle choices. Sharing the responsibility of reducing risks for illness or for managing chronic illness, and helping patients make informed choices about their diagnostic or therapeutic options are all part of sharing responsibility. And sharing responsibility should help strengthen the connection.

attending to the world - I remember learning in my first few days of medical school that the hallmark feature of any true professional—perhaps especially physicians—is the commitment to put the interests our patients ahead of our own. I think that's really what service is about. If all we do is exchange our professional skills for money, then we are more like tradesmen. I hope we don't lose our profession's long-standing commitment to put the interests of our patients above our own in critical situations, and give a little more of ourselves. I believe there is some degree of self-sacrifice required if we want to call ourselves true professionals and caring physicians.

uplifting the medically underserved - I think society has, by and large, answered this question over the last 30 or 40 years. Most of us believe that access to appropriate healthcare services should be an essential human right. No one should have to lose their eyesight to a preventable or readily manageable illness, or die of appendicitis for lack of access to care.

That said, I don't think we have the luxury of saying we will provide anything and everything that is available medically as an inherent right without regard to the cost and potential benefit. For example, what should we do when there is an extraordinarily expensive treatment that has an exceedingly poor chance of prolonging life of reasonable quality? These are questions that will become even more challenging as the chronic illnesses that accompany an aging population become more prevalent. In order to provide effective access to appropriate care as our population ages and physician/population ratios shrink, we will need to work with more non-physician healthcare professionals in the diagnosis and management of many routine acute and chronic illnesses. And yes, I would be fine with having a capable and conscientious non-physician health professional such as a nurse practitioner or physician assistant help manage a routine acute or chronic illness for me or one of my family members.

But how we successfully provide appropriate access to all finally depends on our ability to improve and transform the system. Determining what's appropriate is something we as physicians can, and should, help resolve within our society.

a life apart - Feeling sadness is part of our human experience and evidence of our shared humanity. It's been part of my experience over many years of practice in caring for patients with urologic cancers. I've often had to share difficult news with people—news that personally saddens me. And I don't feel that I'm diminished in their eyes by showing that I care. I don't think showing some emotion hurts a physician's professional image, because part of being a doctor is showing that we do care about people as individuals, and don't see them as simply another diagnosis. That said, we need to not be so overcome emotionally that it interferes with our objectivity in caring for a patient or others for whom we have responsibility. We need to cultivate resiliency. I'm not a medical oncologist who is dealing with death and dying every day. Those specialists need really special adaptive skills. For some physicians who deal with very difficult things on a daily basis, they may have to develop stronger emotional resilience, and perhaps a thicker skin, to deal with the daily challenges. For most of us, though, who aren't immersed in death and dying every day, we ought to be able to appropriately mourn. Mourning is important, and I think it's really important to appropriately show that to medical students and residents. I remember when I was a surgery resident, the doctors I respected most were those who you could tell had a sincere emotional connection with their patients, where you could see they were sincerely disappointed by the bad news that sometimes comes. I didn't feel much connection at all to physicians who seemed more machine-like in their relationships with patients.

a loving smile - I think we need to be bonded to our patients through shared trust, shared openness, and mutual respect. And it really has to work both ways. I've had patients who just couldn't relate to me. Everything I'd say seemed to be met with skepticism. I've had rare situations where it seemed obvious there probably wasn't going to be the good patient-doctor relationship necessary for optimal management of a complex or serious illness. My way of dealing with this has been to say: "It seems like we haven't really connected on a level beyond the most basic language. Do you feel that way?" And sometimes they would say something along the lines of, "Well, I think you're arrogant or not very smart." I liked to get these feelings out in the open. My response would be: "It's important for you to feel like you can have trust and openness with your doctor," and I would suggest another doctor who might better fit their style. Sometimes, they would say "I didn't mean it to come out that way," and we'd get back on the right track. In other cases they chose to leave and receive care elsewhere. We need to recognize that whether it's called a bond or trust, when we're dealing with serious problems people need to feel good about their doctors and how we're helping them. This is not to say we need to become close friends with our patients, only that we develop a relationship of mutual trust.

There's another important consideration when it comes to friendship with patients. When I was a surgery resident in my second year, one of the senior surgeons called to tell me that someone was about to be admitted to our service whom I would recognize because he was a well-known member of the faculty at the medical school. I said, "Well ok, I'll be sure to take good care of him." The attending said, "Actually, I want you to treat him no differently than you treat everybody else." He told me that once we start treating people differently because they are our friends or colleagues or VIPs, we start to make judgments that aren't objective. When we do that, the odds become pretty good that they will actually have a less positive outcome. This is a principle that I've always remembered and followed, and one that I've tried to pass along to medical students and residents over the years.

a story - Training as a surgeon, I was focused so strongly on clinical outcomes and evidenced-based practices, and of course really trying to develop excellent surgical technique, that initially I underestimated the importance of the connection we make with people. Not that I think I wasn't warm or friendly or that I didn't care about others. I just underestimated the difference I could make beyond my technical skills. I became very aware of that throughout my practice. In one case, after about 10 years, I had a patient referred to me with a very large renal cell carcinoma that required extensive surgery to resect the tumor. Our team did the surgery and there was very little blood loss, and I remember we were pleased with how the procedure had gone. I also remember talking to the patient's wife and their two children, who were probably ages 10 and 12 at the time. "Good news. Surgery went very well," I told them. I remember feeling really good about myself. We had completed a challenging case, and I thought this man was going to recover. But about a year later, he returned with some weight loss and nausea, and a CT scan showed recurrent disease. I was extremely disappointed. He died about 12 months after that.

His children were still young, and I felt like a failure. I wished that I could have done something more to help.

About a decade later, I was waiting for the elevator near my office and saw a young woman looking intently at me. She said, "Aren't you Dr. Sorenson?" She told me her name and said: "You took care of our Dad." I instantly remembered this young woman who had been about 12 at the time. I told her, "I do remember your Dad and I'm really sorry about his passing." She said, "You made a really big difference for our family." I was a little taken aback. She said: "It was a hard thing for all of us, but we all felt like you were someone who really cared about him and did everything that could be done." Then she gave me a hug.

I think as young medical students, we can get so focused on the technical skills we need to perform that we forget we can make a huge difference for people who are going through some of the hardest times of their lives by showing them that we care about them. Sometimes we just can't cure them, but we can always care for and about them. Intermountain Healthcare's tagline is "Healing for Life". When that line was first proposed to me I resisted it, knowing we can't always cure people. But as I thought more deeply about it, I realized that though we can't always offer a cure, healing involves something that goes beyond treatment and curing. Some of the patients with whom I've developed the closest relationships have been those I couldn't cure, but for whom I had the privilege of helping them as much as I could through a difficult crossroad in their life.

a lens into your life - I still get back to the operating room a number of times each month. These are some of my favorite days at work. What I love about surgery is the opportunity—when you have some big case coming up the next day, even if you have done it many times before—to rehearse in your mind what you're going to do, and then having the satisfaction when you're finished of knowing that it went well. I always like to finish a big operation by taking a moment with the team. We talk about what went well and what we might do better next time. That feeling of accomplishment with a team of people is pretty special. I enjoy my administrative responsibilities at Intermountain, especially the opportunity of working with very bright and dedicated people. But the thing I miss most as CEO is that I don't have the long-term patient interactions I used to. Some of the best rewards in medicine for me are the long-term relationships and personal affection that develop when we provide care to a patient.

On the administrative side, the thing that makes my best days are when I'm out there with our staff who provide care and when they say, "You know, we've been able to use this information, or this Intermountain process, to improve our outcomes in this particular way. Thanks for letting us be a part of this." To me, medicine is the ultimate team sport. Historically, it may have been drilled into us that the physician is the captain of the ship. Yet, now we know that it's just way too complex for one person to figure it all out by himself or herself. A team of engaged people working together consistently leads to much better outcomes and makes our profession far more fulfilling.

Donna Ferriero

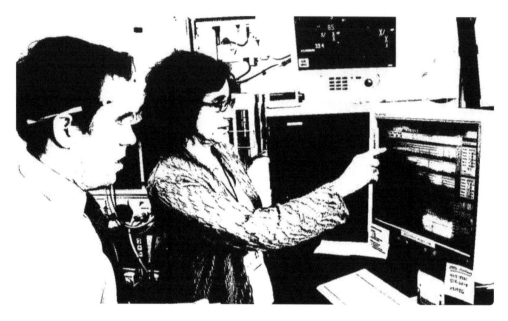

Donna M. Ferriero M.D. is W.H. And Marie Wattis Distinguished Professor and Chair of the University of California, San Francisco, Department of Pediatrics, and Physician-in-Chief of UCSF Benioff Children's Hospital.

our white coat – The white coat, I will argue today, is an excellent example of a traditional symbol needing rethinking. How do doctors define themselves, present themselves as physicians and healers without this symbol? Perhaps we can project our empathy, compassion, altruism, and commitment to medical expertise by our actions and words, rather than our couture. The primacy of the patient will be easier to understand if we don't set ourselves apart with uniforms that distinguish us. Do white coats create a sense of entitlement to trust and respect that is unhealthy and in turn may foster an elitism that separates patient from caregiver?

attending to the world - Physicians must be agents of change. As our health care environment undergoes change (for the better we hope), physicians must possess the values, the experiences, and the talents to create and improve the future of healthcare. The attending physician must teach these values as well as serve, and inform the future caregivers and patients that this service is critical to the wellbeing of all.

a loving smile - As a physician, my greatest pleasure comes from connecting with others. I believe that one must be able to touch another human being, not just as part of a physical examination, but in a tender, caring way-with words, actions, and genuine emotion.

a life apart - It is always okay to feel sad about loss, about needless suffering. Moving forward involves a partnership with those experiencing loss and suffering. This is where the bond between patient and provider becomes strengthened.

a story - One of the sad parts of being a pediatrician is that our patients grow up and leave our practices. One patient of mine who had very difficult seizures to treat as a child, and was hard to convince to be compliant with medications as a teenager, recently contacted me. He is now married, has taught himself to be a metal worker, and makes jewelry. He brought me a bracelet that he made and told me that my persistence convinced him that he needed to take better care of himself.

a lens - *(Editor's note: The image is on Dr. Ferriero's cover page).*

Edward Benz

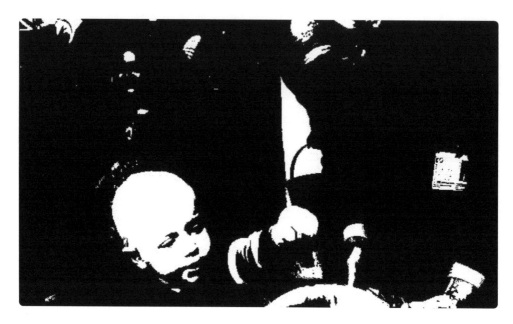

Edward Benz M.D. is President and CEO of The Dana Farber Cancer Center at Harvard Medical School.

our white coat - Because I am now President of the Institute, I am somewhat reflecting on my past experiences when I could give more direct care to patients. As I age and observe more and more clinical experiences I think increasingly that the best way for a patient and a provider to approach their relationship is as a partnership. The physician has the knowledge, expertise, and access to all the resources that are needed from a clinical perspective, but the patient really brings a tremendous amount to the care-giving as well as to the care-receiving process. The communication must be a two way street. Patients who have the most positive experience are the patients who are very active participants in their care. In that sense, they too are wearing the white coat.

attending to the world - In virtually every sense of the word, an attending physician is serving a number of human beings. Certainly you are serving the patient who trusts you with his or her care. You are there to serve the patients clinically, to alleviate pains that come from the impact of the condition on his or her life and the lives of their family members. You are also there to serve the learners who are there as a part of their training. They trust you with how to become competent in becoming an expert and in living by the values that will determine how they will provide care when their training is finished. In every process, I think you are serving multiple human beings in your role as an attending physician. It is very important to remember that even if you are on a so-called teaching service, and might be removed from primary care responsibilities, you are serving the creation of a team atmosphere around the patient with all of the healthcare professionals and supporting personnel.

uplifting the medically underserved - With regard to access to healthcare as a basic human right, that question probably belongs to those who trained in divinity school as well as those who trained in constitutional law. In the United States, a country that has the resources to provide healthcare to everyone, access to a competent physician should be everyone's right, and that is true if you are in any of the advanced societies where it is possible to do so. In that context, it is a right that a member of that particular society has. More broadly, if you look at the rest of the world, those individuals should also have an expectation that they should have a physician. I am not sure how you can define how that plays out in different societies that have differ-

ent value systems. If the resources are there, everyone should have the right to a physician, and if the resources are not there then they should be created. In my own role in dealing with this issue, I perhaps am less able to make an impact as an individual physician other than that I will choose to see anyone who chooses to see me. In my role as CEO of a cancer institute, I make sure that we invest in, support and advocate for research in disparities, which will hopefully lead to better interventions that will decrease disparities in the long term. We engage in outreach programs that try to address directly additional ways for disadvantaged populations to access us. We invest in advocacy to ensure that everybody who has some role in creating or regulating those resources—at the state, local, and federal level—is doing a proper job of trying to address disparities.

a loving smile - The issue of showing emotion is appropriate. One has to be a little bit more careful not to be completely unrestrained, because as an attending physician you have to maintain some degree of equanimity. If you fall completely apart, then you are modeling that everyone should fall completely apart when those who depend on and work with you really need for you to have your act together enough to support the patient and his or her family. I don't think you can be completely buttoned down, but there is some modulation for the emotional response you are inclined to have, when you are responsible for being able to support others. You can have a major emotional meltdown when you are by yourself or with other people, in your personal life.

I think that it is important to emphasize that it is always appropriate to form a bond with a patient. I worry a little about some people's notion of bonding with a patient, because of variation in what that might mean. You can't have a solely "professional" relationship like financial consultants or other service professionals might maintain. At the same time, I will say that you can go too far at times with that bonding. Part of your role as a physician is to be able to step back at times, and say I won't be dispassionate but I need to make decisions that require an objective perspective that may be too difficult if I get too emotionally invested. It is one of those very difficult things that you do learn from experience. Part of your responsibility is to provide perspective and objectivity. Yet, if you don't feel some connection, you are going to have an awfully hard time in understanding where the patient is coming from. If you don't understand that, you cannot make the best decision. You cannot protect yourself from one extreme by going to the other.

a life apart - It is always appropriate to feel sad. On some level, if you don't feel sadness at a patient's passing or when having to deliver the news that things are not going to go well, you probably haven't connected either with the patient or with yourself adequately. It is appropriate to feel sadness when the situation is one in which any reasonable person would feel sad. Paradoxically, some of the times I have felt sad

have also been when patients have done quite well. It means saying goodbye to them, saying goodbye for a good reason, but feeling some loss of your role in their lives because they don't need you any more. It feels like saying goodbye to a friend or family member. It made me happy that they were doing well but nostalgic for the relationship. I remember taking care of babies that only weighed seven hundred grams until they graduated to a regular nursery. This was a moment of clear happiness and – on the other hand – clear sadness. It is thus completely appropriate to feel sadness. If you don't, you are fooling yourself, or you really have detached yourself too much from your patients to be a good physician.

a story - "Harriet" (name changed) presented to me with anemia, when I was a mid-career faculty member at Yale University School of Medicine. When she and her husband arrived, I could sense almost instantly that she and her husband had a very troubled relationship. From her past history it was clear that she was constantly developing symptoms and looking for secondary gain or just enough attention from her husband to try to hang onto their relationship. I looked at the slides that her referring doctor had sent and it was immediately apparent that she had multiple melanoma. I had to tell her that and, instead of a look of devastation, the look on her face was triumphant. She told her husband, "See, I told you I was sick." It took me multiple visits to work with her and her husband on the realities of what she was facing and the way to deal with the treatment. She actually ended up doing quite well for a number of years. She had what we then called smoldering melanoma. We had seemed to develop a good relationship, but she was a very fearful woman underneath all of that. I wouldn't have classified her husband as terribly understanding and/or supportive. We were working on our schedule of medications, and she kept objecting to every potential schedule. She seemed to more flexibility, yet, with each increasingly flexible proposal she became more upset. I asked her if there was something she wasn't telling me that I could help her with, because I had built up a strong relationship and it seemed no matter what I suggested - even when I included more flexibility - she wanted to have a fight with me. She then told me that if she didn't fight, she was going to die, because some doctor had told her that if she didn't fight with her physician, she was not advocating well enough for herself. We worked through all of that. I told her, "I'm not quite sure that is what they meant. I think this medication is helping you. But, if you want me to fight, ok, I hereby order you to take this medication next week." She seemed stunned but pleased! She lived another five years with her melanoma. She lived the last few months at home with hospice care. She ended up dying on Christmas Day, when there was no coroner available. I had to make a house call and pronounce her dead. When I was leaving, I was handed a little present from her daughter that was under the Christmas tree, intended, I supposed, for when I would have

stopped in to see her after the New Year. It was a little framed note from her that said, "Thank you for fighting with me." So you never quite know what is going on in a patient's heart and soul and mind, and how what you're doing is impacting what they view as your care. It speaks to the need to try incredibly hard to have that meaningful personal connection.

Erika Goldstein

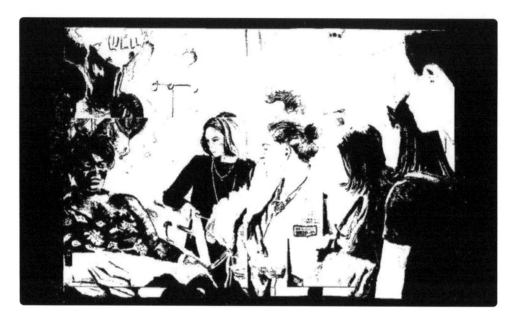

Erika Goldstein, M.D. is Dean for the Colleges at the University of Washington School of Medicine.

our white coat - The challenge of the coat is that it is important to not separate physicians from patients. At the same time, you have special knowledge that they don't have. There are certain settings in our community where physicians don't wear white coats to try to minimize the distance between doctors and patients. I wear a white coat frankly because I need the pockets. I work in a county hospital in the out-patient setting, and most of the patients are economically and socially disadvantaged. I once heard a patient saying to one of our nursing assistants that even though she was poor, she really appreciated that the doctors in our clinic in particular wore a white coat. It meant to her that she was being valued in the same way and respected in the same way as patients who had more resources. It formalized a relationship, which was important.

attending to the world - Attending is primarily used in the educational setting. Doctors in practice don't usually talk about themselves as Attendings. Attending is part of the medical education hierarchy, we all attend to our patients, and in a teaching setting, physicians attend to their students as well, in ways that hopefully model the really important responsibilities of caring for patients and the gift of taking care of patients.

a loving smile - That's one of the things that students observe, though it's a very private thing that happens between doctor and patient. With experienced clinicians, the bond forms very quickly, it's one of the things that the students get to see. They see that it's not too difficult to obtain. The observer learns to be a physician, in part by learning to maintain genuineness.

a story - This is one of my favorite stories. I have been in practice for 32 years. I have been teaching for about 25 of those years. It is my favorite story in my country's hospital. I was working with a group of students at the bedside, a group of second year students. The patient had been hospitalized with a foot fracture and sang in a church choir. She was telling us about how these two young men who had been enthusiastically rolling the piano, rolled it over her foot. In the course of receiving treatment, she developed a pulmonary embolism. She ended up in the intensive care unit. Her voice was really important to her, and she was worried about intubation and the effect it would have on her vocal coords. She told a student this and he was telling his colleagues. They agreed that nurses

would watch her overnight, and if her oxygen stayed above a certain level, they wouldn't intubate her.

While she was on the mend, she never required intubation and we met her after she was discharged from the intensive care unit and back on the Medicine floor. We were adjusting her Coumadin. Talking with her about this was very moving because it had been really important to her. One of my other students had been smiling at her and asked, "Are we going to get a sample?" The patient next to her had a great smile, almost all of our rooms have two beds. She just started singing two A cappella gospel songs, and I had tears in my eyes. The students and nurses all clustered around the door, and the woman just sung her heart out.

I always take our second year students one morning a week to do a complete history and physical. They then present their findings to their colleagues. I always say to the patient, here are six students who are going to be starting clinical training, what do you have to tell them about being a good doctor? I said to the vocalist, you already gave us such a tremendous gift, any thoughts on what would make a good doctor?

Her minister had spent much of the night next to her bed, praying that she would not require intubation. She picked up a Bible and turned to a section that read, "Consider the lilies in the field. They don't labor and spin. They're so grounded to the earth. They just lean with the wind." The message was that you have to take care of yourself and let others take care of you so you can take care of others. It remains one of my favorite stories. What you get back from your patients captures the notion that patients are our best teachers.

Ironically, there happened to be a staff-member doing a report with us that day. He took a photograph and later gave it to her. He also created a painting, and that's what they gave me when I stepped away from my two-year sequence of the clinical course, a course I had chaired for twenty years. Most of the medical students didn't know the story of the photograph, most graduated six to seven years ago. It is amazing that they choose that picture to use for the basis of the painting that hangs on the wall of my office. It is absolutely the most important and moving to me.

a lens - I've been at this for a while. No two days are alike. There is far too much time in front of the computer, one month of full four weeks on the wards, which I have to say is probably my favorite. It combines both amazing opportunities for patient care and also the chance to be part of a regular team of care. A lot of my days now are spent in meetings; computers are my absolutely least favorite. The best days are days spent with students and patients together. We may have a picture of the painting, the woman sitting in her bed. It is pretty amazing, in a funny way he made it up of a lot of refracted pictures, embodying the complexity of what we do. I really do intensely dislike what technology has done to interactions between patient and doctor; what has remained constant is the human relationship, the physician-patient relationship, the teacher-learner relationship. Those are the essential fundamentals which never change. What really draws people into medicine, sustains people in medicine, sustains teachers of medicine, and is a gift to both patients and students are these relationships.

Eric Klein

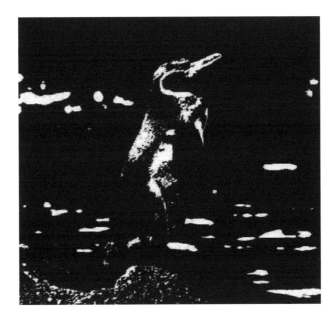

Eric Klein M.D. is Chairman at the Glickman Urological Institute and the Cleveland Clinic.

our white coat - I always thought that the white coat acted as a barrier between patient and physician. In one sense, the white coat makes the physician the expert and identifies him or her as the focal point. In another sense, it belongs to the patient, in a way that allows them to identify the source of the information and choose to accept the treatment they are seeking. My philosophy has always been to see their disease or problem through their own eyes and connect with them on a human level; to do my best to be on an equal basis with them; and to show them that we are partners in healing. I never want to see myself and my patients as separate. The white coat can separate and be a barrier between doctor and patient, and because of this I often don't wear a white coat when I see patients in my office or when I round. I think it helps brand me in the eyes of my patients as a regular person and allows me to relate to them on a more open and human level. It creates a sense of commonality, as opposed to viewing me as an expert who is a separate entity.

Regarding my particular practice, I focus primarily on prostate cancer and the multiple treatment choices with roughly equal outcomes. My patients and I are both healers in a sense that we have a significant degree of shared decision making. My job is to educate the patient on what the options are and not guide them to necessarily what I think the best option may be. Instead, it is my duty to educate them in a manner that helps them avoid making a mistake. Sometimes there are circumstances with three or four quality care options. One patient might want to avoid the hassle of specific side effects from a certain option, and another might want to avoid treatment entirely on a low-grade cancer, which is something that is reasonable and which I respect. The ultimate goal is to have the patient pick the choice that makes them feel most comfortable. In that way, we are shared healers.

attending to the world - There are a number of levels to this question, what it means to attend to the world. One way is to endeavor to connect to patients at a very human level. You want to be seen as a friend or co-equal whose expertise happens to be in medicine, as opposed to an auto-repair person or tax professional. In a more literal way, at my Institute at the Cleveland Clinic, we've seen people from more than 70 countries around the world in just the last several years. In a bigger way, I like to think about this concept in the context of making observations and sharing patient outcomes through the medical education process, and

through publishing in the medical literature. A defining moment for me in my career – that "aha" moment – was when I first started my practice. I was doing major surgery to remove the prostate, yet the functional outcomes weren't terrific, and it took patients several months to regain urinary control after surgery. We didn't really understand the anatomy clearly and based on the work of others I made some modifications to the surgical procedure. The very first paper I submitted, in 1991, had some observations on minor alterations that resulted in much earlier return to control for about sixty patients. It was a pretty significant advance, allowing patients to regain urinary control in a matter of weeks as opposed to a number of months. About a year later, I was at a major urological meeting in San Diego. Someone I hadn't met before approached me and said, "Dr. Klein, I want to thank you for publishing that paper on the surgical technique of radical prostatectomy.," in a very heartfelt way. Before I read your paper, I didn't understand the anatomy, and now that I've read the article and understood it my patients are doing much, much better." I was overwhelmed. Being speechless is usually a rare thing for me, and because I was so moved by the power of publishing on a small number of patients – I was truly speechless. The possibility to truly change the outcomes for many more patients, those I will never operate upon, people I will never see or meet or know existed, struck me. Publishing scientific observations multiplies the way that we are able to have an impact. It just seems extraordinary to me to be able to multiply the contributions we make. This is the power of anyone who is attuned to observation, who records processes and results well, to change lives in a meaningful way for others that you actually never see as patients.

uplifting the medically underserved - It is my belief that having access to good quality medical care is a basic human right. It is a matter of how does one influence a political system in whatever circumstance one lives in. Compared to the rights to have freedom of speech, group defense etc., I'm not sure I'm philosophically trained to understand nor am I sure I can give you a great answer to this. The human right and political systems should find a way to get everyone the care that they need. Although I do not have a direct role in pursuing health equity, we do provide access to the underserved population and the local population by virtue of working at a large academic medical center. To the extent that patients have urological needs, I do everything I can to heal them. I have colleagues who have a bigger role in this and have taken time out of their practice to share their expertise. They have helped patients, particularly in Africa, where fistulas result in young women having serious gynecological issues that make them social pariahs until they are fixed. Some of my colleagues donate their time, and I feel I help facilitate this. Prostate cancer is not one of the biggest day-to-day problems of the medically underserved – so many other medical specialists may play a more direct role. Yet, I try to do everything I can as Chair. We make room for all of our residents and some of our attending staff who do medical missionary activities to take time off for this type of work.

a loving smile - I think a smile is absolutely essential to be the most effective physician. You have to see the problem from the patient's eyes, and that requires a degree of personal bonding. When I see a new patient in the clinic, I have to find something that bonds me with them that is outside of my expertise as a clinician and outside of the problem that theya re seeking advice for. If they are visiting with their spouse, I'll ask them how many children they have, I will tell them about my family. If they are wearing a piece of clothing that indicates they are a fan of a particular team, I will pick up on that.

I saw a patient whose name sounded vaguely familiar. I thought, "That sounds like a public figure." I recognized him, it turned out that he was an astronaut in the NASA program. We talked about that for 10 minutes before we talked about his medical problems. With another patient, my resident picked up that he was a musician. I started asking him about his musical career and learned he was a guitarist from a locally famous group outside of Cleveland, which was fairly prominent in the 1970s. He gave me a bunch of CDs including a concert that they played at Carnegie Hall. I listened to his CD on the car ride home, and it was absolutely awesome Whenever I come out of the room, what I always tell my resident is to put the patient in the context of their own life and to not miss out on the wonderful experience that the patient is trying to live. When they go in, I ask that they please not focus the entire time on the patient's medical condition. It distracts patients from their medical problem and makes them feel like their doctor is human too. It relates to my preference for the lack of a white coat. It creates an environment for the patients to connect to you as another person, and I have heard many wonderful stories as a result of this. One of the other things I do that I find important is that I interview residency and fellowship candidates. I always ask them about the most challenging thing in their lives professionally and personally. They open up about the experiences and hardships in their lives. One guy said his most recent challenge was climbing Mt. Kilimanjaro, and I thought that was pretty cool. I've found the ability to discuss one's own challenges in life can be a very meaningful part of connecting with patients.

a life apart - One of my favorite stories is a story about something that made me very sad. It was when I was an intern, I was sad to begin with because I was on call for Christmas Day, which happens to be my birthday. This was in the era before we had a well-defined discipline called palliative care. I was taking care of an old woman who had metastatic cancer. It was a situation in which I had very little prior experience, and the emotional needs of the patient and family were great. None of us were prepared to appropriately comfort her. She had been in the hospital for weeks and weeks and did not respond to the therapies we attempted. She had a devoted sister who spent hours with her each day, sitting by her, and holding her hand. Her sister's one wish in life was to be with the patients when she died. Christmas came. I can't help but choke up telling you this story, even though it was 30 years ago. It was noon on Christmas Day, and while she was very ill, we did not think she would die that day and encouraged her sister to go home for Christmas dinner. We assured her sister that the patient wouldn't die when she was gone; sadly she died while her sister was at Christmas dinner, and we had to call her tell her that. That is the saddest thing that has ever happened in my medical career, maybe even my entire life. Those of us who were taking care of her, trainees and otherwise, sat there and cried because it made us realize that our best intentions in medicine sometimes are unsuccessful. We have to always be aware of that.

I think we have seen a change in the expectation about trainees who come to medicine, and it seems to be a generational issue. We see some trainees who view medicine as a job rather than a career, they become a little overly focused on becoming great technicians rather than having a global view and strong knowledge base in medicine. I recently had a young medical student rotate with me, and we were talking about this issue. One of my mantras for everyone is that they need to read the medical literature more. He said, "That doesn't resonate with my generation. We are more about carrying tablets around and looking up information on the web as needed." I think that to really be a complete physician, you really need a good knowledge base, to be able to make connections about things you would otherwise be unable to make. You might not put one with the other if you look up information only on a need-to-know basis.

a story - The story I like most is the one about the guy who thanked me for publishing that article, and I think young people find that inspiring. That is the one I would use here too. But while I would like to bring additional attention to that one, I will tell you one other that is a humbling story as well. I use this for humor and so forth. When my wife and I moved to Cleveland and started our careers, we got a Labrador puppy whose name was Opus. He was incredibly well known by all our neighbors. We got to know our neighbors through him. He plays a prominent part in this story, which starts here: Early in my career, I operated on a locally prominent person. He asked me to do a press conference and tell people how important PSA screening was. My ego got the better of me, and I started to say, "Wow, this is so wonderful that I get to do this, this is going to make me famous, etc." Well, the press conference only lasted about 30 seconds and was a complete bust. The local media was not interested, the story was all good news, and it was over. I was really disappointed, and the next day I was in the operating room and a friend came up to me and said in a very animated way, "My family and I were having dinner last night, and your face came on the screen, and my daughter got very excited and said "Look, there's Opus's Dad!" This helped me keep things in perspective –it really emphasized for me that being substantive was more important than being a celebrity.

a lens into your life - I have an incredibly rich and rewarding professional life that has a lot of important roles for me to play. I am Chairman of a 300-person institute. I am an educator for residents and fellows, a surgeon, an academician, a little bit of a scientist, and a journal editor. I am responsible for financial endeavors, a mentor to many people, a marketer, and a businessman – all of those things. One of the things I really enjoy about my life is that no two days are the same because of the diversity of roles. When I was just a physician for 20 years, you could name any day and any hour, and I could tell you what I'll be doing. Thursday afternoon at four o'clock next week, I'll be in the operating room. Six months from now, Thursday at 4 o'clock, I'll be in the operating room. Once I became Institute Chair, all those other roles went out the window. My life gained an unpredictable rhythm to it, and it gives me chances to drive medicine forward while at the same time it challenges me to be excellent in more ways than I can count. There's one additional role that is why I am still going. I get to be a father and husband seven days a week – I don't think it could get any better than that. I really don't think so.

Eugene Washington

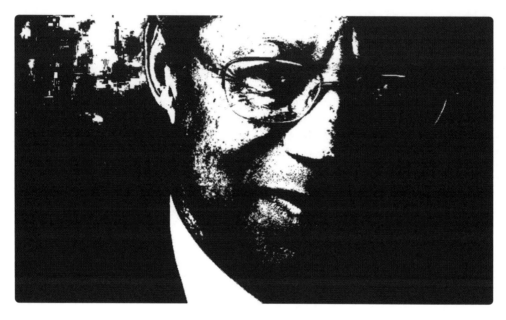

A. Eugene Washington M.D. is Dean of the David Geffen School of Medicine and Vice Chancellor for Health Sciences at the University of California, Los Angeles.

our white coat - The white coat, for me, is really a symbol. While it was originally connected to hygiene, in terms of the color itself, the coat is now a symbol of hope and expectation - and this goes both ways, for the patient as well as for the provider. With the white coat on, there's both expectations that we have and there's expectations that the patients have. Those expec-

tations and hopes bind us together with the view that there's a partnership formed through the symbol of this white coat. It's also a symbol of respect. It's in many ways, depending on the setting, a symbol of the future of medicine from our perspective because the young doctors, who don these coats at their white coat ceremony, represent the future of the discipline.

attending to the world - Empathy is arguably the most important requisite for being a successful physician. That doesn't mean that the physician has to experience every disease or condition. But it does mean that the physician has made a diligent effort to try to walk in the shoes of every patient he treats.

a loving smile - A loving smile is critical. It welcomes the patient in a warm and nurturing way and helps to encourage the patient to relax, be open. Just through its physical nature, a smile says "I want to help."

a life apart - I feel like you can't define when it is appropriate to feel sad, you know it. I think we know it. I don't think it's appropriate to come up with a definition of when to feel sad because it is a reflection of who we are and is dependent on the circumstances. When you're sad, that's the threshold point, you might not want to be sad - but it's there.

When I'm sad, people around me tend to notice. First of all, I'm quiet. When I'm sad, I'm introspective and that's not usually my nature. In general, I'm outwardly oriented and I've got a pretty smiley demeanor. It's just who I am. I deal with sadness with a sort of taciturnity. I go inward and become quiet because I'm internally processing and thinking, at least until I can get to a moment of solitude without anyone around me. For me to eventually get over it, I've got to have some space where I can really reflect on what this means for me, not just in this moment, but what it means for me in the context of medicine. I reflect on what I might do differently or how I might find even more engagement, in terms of what I do in medicine, to help me feel that even in moments like this there is

some meaning. These moments remind you that life is still there and you have to get back in even more charged up than before.

I believe it's absolutely appropriate to show emotion in front of trainees. I think that that's a part of their training, to be reminded that in medicine, we're human, and as humans we experience pain and we experience the emotions of people we've connected with. There are multiple dimensions to the interaction with patients and their family. There are multiple individuals and personalities involved. People deal with that environment in different ways. I wouldn't expect everyone on my team to be calibrated on the same emotional level. We all deal with sadness and setbacks in different ways as a function of who we are, how we've been raised and partly, our cultural experiences. There is certainly a standard of respect that needs to be there and a standard of compassion that needs to be exhibited in the way you behave and the way you treat colleagues as well as patients. As leader of a team in particular, we have a responsibility to work to connect the team so that everyone is comfortable expressing themselves in a way that is respectful but also most natural for who they each are.

a story - When I was a house staff, my worst rotation was unquestionably in oncology. First of all, it was a brutal rotation in terms of hours. Second, we had a chief resident who I thought was out of her mind. In fact, I went to complain to the chair of the department even though I was only a first year. I thought that this person was someone out of a textbook as psychotic. He told me, "You know she's not really that bad when she takes her medication," confirming what I thought. That's the setting. There were two attending doctors. One of them was like a bull in a china shop. The other eventually became the chair of OBGYN at UC Davis but at the time he was just a fellow in oncology. One day there was a family, their mother was dying. And I tear up just thinking about this. As the family was gathered around the mother, we entered the room. The oncology fellow didn't simply shake her hand, but instinctively, he dropped down on one knee and grabbed her hand just as gently as you could imagine and just held it. In that moment, if I had any doubts about the discipline, about what I wanted to be like in medicine, in terms of a physician – they were gone. I can still see Lloyd Smith on one knee with a hand gently soothing. That's what medicine is about.

And you teach that by example, through trying to expose as many of our students to faculty and residents with that natural ability. You want those "Lloyd Smith's" to have as much exposure to the students as possible. That's why I like recognizing these people, through awards like the Arnold P. Gold Humanism award. It's why I have participated in both Service Minded Physicians editions. That's why I like the fact that we have we have a new vice dean who studied in education and bioethics; I can see his commitment to students. It's not something we can test for, per se. When I'm asked 'what's the most important, innate quality for the best physi-

cians?' – It is empathy. Having the knowledge is great and necessary but you have to be able to feel it, to put yourself there.

a lens into your life - My best days are when I'm with the future leaders of tomorrow. When I think of my best days, the days I go home and I greet my wife with a big smile, it's because I just met a student with a great idea. There's an organization called the California C5 Association of Los Angeles. The "C5" refers to going to college within 5 years. It's a program that was funded early on by the former president of Coca-Cola. They formed a cohort of 8th-12th grade students from inner city schools across the LA area. The organization developed a curriculum, including academic enrichment such as going out and meeting with different professionals. Someone introduced them to me a couple years ago, and I've been involved ever since. Just two weeks ago I hosted a group of six students. They have lunch with me and we just talk. We walk up to the Ronald Reagan Hospital, tour around various labs, like Dr. Yang's and I introduce them to medical students in the hallway. Not all of them are going into medicine, some of them are thinking about other careers, but they are the future. That is one of the most important contributions that I make and it's how I honor all the people who have generously given their time to me.

Gary Gottlieb

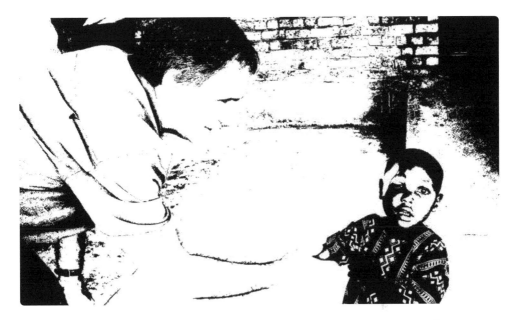

Gary Gottlieb M.D. is President and CEO of Partners Healthcare. Partners Healthcare is the collegium of the Harvard University School of Medicine teaching hospitals.

our white coat - My perspective is that caring for patients is an extraordinary privilege. Any care plan that is going to be successful requires the patient, his or her family, and other important people in his or her life to be at the center of it. The physician and the healthcare system are only parts to the plan. Patients teach us about empathy, about how to connect in a way

that we can do the most good. They teach us how to understand their experience, the human condition, and what kinds of interventions might be appropriate for us to implement together. They teach us not to just cure specific diseases, but also to make improvements overall to that individual's well being and ultimately their life. As we continue to develop the healthcare system for the future, we need to move away from a system that is centered on providers, and create one that is centered upon patients and their families. In doing so, we can create outcomes that are meaningful for each patient and that improve the quality of life from the perspective of the individual person and his or her family.

attending to the world - I believe that every aspect of being a physician is a commitment to a broad-based mission that is to improve the human condition in the patients we care for. The focus of every great physician's activity is to ease pain, to cure illness, and to do it in a way that is connected to an individual patient's circumstances and the breadth of their needs. As leaders, we need to be committed to improving the human condition globally. That means creating accessible healthcare as well as food stability, housing stability, and all that we do as stewards of the human condition.

uplifting the medically underserved - I believe that healthcare is a right and not a privilege. I believe it is a basic civil right and that ensuring access to great healthcare through skilled professionals and exceptional institutions is a matter of social justice. I think health equity is one of the great measures of being able to meet such an objective. Every person, regardless of financial means or geography, needs to have access to excellent healthcare and state-of-the-art care in the same way that they need access to adequate housing and nutrition.

a loving smile - I think it is always appropriate to create a bond with patients in medicine. That bond has to be appropriate for the clinical circumstances. It has to respect the boundaries of privacy and the nature of the professional relationship between the patient and the physician. There should be a connection for the patient to feel that the physician is being thoughtful and empathetic so that the patient can depend upon the physician to be responsible to his or her breadth of medical needs. Patients need to create a bond with physicians in order for there to be trust.

a life apart - I think it is appropriate to be saddened when one sees someone suffer a loss. When one empathizes with the experience of loss it makes that person a better doctor, a nurse or care provider. It is appropriate for a leader to be sad when one sees failure in the healthcare system or in the delivery of the mission and greater good to which we are all committed. I think it is appropriate for one to show emotional responses to trainees so that they understand that they have the freedom to experience emotion in association with the challenges of providing healthcare. Even in the situations that require the utmost caution and professionalism, it is still important that one shows enough emotion to demonstrate that one is empathetic to each individual patient.

a story - I think that most of the stories that have inspired me are the stories of heroism of patients and the pain and challenge that they have to suffer in order to care for themselves and their families. When patients overcome uncertainty, their heroism inspires me to work as

hard as I possibly can to find solutions. I don't
have a special caveat, every patient inspires me.

a lens into your life - I have this great privilege
in my role at Partners HealthCare of being able
to facilitate many more people who are smarter
than I could ever dream to be. People whose
commitment to serving patients, to finding
cures, and to finding solutions to challenges
presented by our healthcare system is breathtaking. The ability to make substantial health improvements on behalf of each of my patients
and the public is the real lens of what keeps me
going, what inspires me. On a personal level,
the centerpiece of my life is my family. Without
that anchor and great strength that I receive
from my wife and kids, my leadership role
would be much too difficult for me, and I would
not be able to do the work that I do.

Jerris Hedges

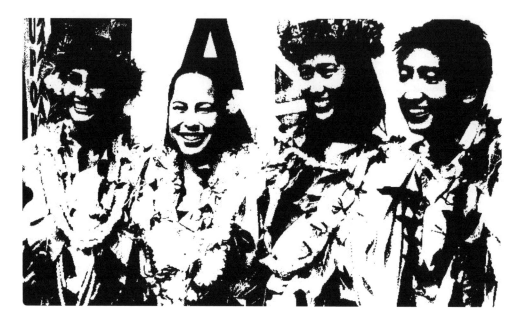

Jerris Hedges, M.D. is Dean of the John A. Burns School of Medicine at the University of Hawaii.

attending to the world - Optimizing health is an active attending service on behalf of our fellow beings. Disease may be slowed or cured at times by intervention with limited knowledge of the patient. Health and well-being can always be improved, but to do so is harder and requires knowing the patient.

our white coat - A white coat is a symbol of our profession, training, and knowledge. It must not be a barrier that obscures understanding. It should be a beacon that draws the patient and family to the doctor for discussion and comfort.

a life apart - Is there a life apart? Being a physician permeates my body and my soul. These days, I am a healer of academic and healthcare systems. A people and all things are in need of healing.

a story - I have treated many patients and impacted and extended many lives. One patient who had a major impact upon me was not one whose life was extended, but rather a yet to be diagnosed cancer patient whose life was to be forever altered by my workup. This person who had been an alcoholic and down on his luck for a decade responded to my touch and chose to turn his life around. He may have only had 1-2 years to live after the diagnosis of metastatic colon cancer, but in his new sober status he could reconnect with his family and humanity. As he said, "Don't feel bad for me as I was dead, but now I live." Life is precious and worthy of celebration, despite the duration.

a loving smile - Children always are the most vulnerable, but the most forgiving. Smiling and playing with the ill child in the emergency department is always a gesture welcomed by the child, parent, and physician.

a lens - Just a few of our Native Hawaiian graduates in their kihei.

Jimmy Hara

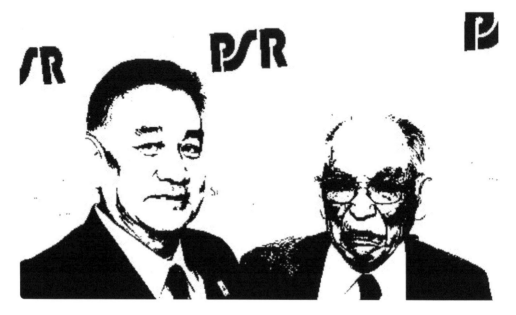

Jimmy Hara M.D. is Professor of Clinical Medicine at the David Geffen School of Medicine at UCLA. Dr. Hara is also Professor of Family Medicine and Associate Dean at Charles Drew University. He is Credentials Chair of the American Board of Family Physicians, and current Los Angeles City Fire Commissioner.

our white coat - I think that the white coat is symbolic. Even in this day and age, the color white implies something plain and clean. And I think it identifies the physician at least in his work frequently. In the old days, on the East Coast, people used to wear bowties and now they are less fashionable. Yet, the color white goes beyond what is fashionable; it is a symbol of what you are all about. It implies that you are something clean and not evil.

I have been a residency director for over 25 years, and I always tell the residents that the patients' problems belong to the patients; the healing is going to be done by the patient. Our role is nothing more than to assist patients to solve their problems, it is their problem. They take an important role in the healing process as the complete healer.

uplifting the medically underserved - Access to care when a patient feels they need the care is obviously a human right. At Kaiser Permanente, we try to do prevention so bad things never happen. So they don't have to come to us because we are taking care of them. The most important thing is to be available when patients really need our services. This is something that every American citizen needs, and every world citizen should be entitled to. I guess that is the reason I have done what I have in my medical career, I feel like everyone really does have the right to healthcare. And I am happy that President Obama is providing access to healthcare to more people. The one problem is here in California, we have a lot of non-citizens and undocumented individuals, and the unfortunate part of the Obamacare plan is that it does not cover them. The reason for that was that he probably wouldn't have been able to push through the whole Obamacare package if he included non-citizens in the mix. A political problem that is a huge problem for California. There are a lot of undocumented individuals who are not yet still given access to appropriate healthcare services.

a story - I am Japanese, and I was born in an internment camp for Japanese Americans. Growing up, I learned about what happened in Hiroshima and Nagasaki. One of my biggest concerns is a nuclear war today. I think a nuclear war is the worst thing that could possibly affect mankind. One of my main motivations has been working to prevent nuclear war in the public health field. My life goal is to make sure that there is never a nuclear bomb detonated ever again anywhere on this planet. In pursuing this goal, I am involved in Physicians for Social Responsibility. I'm on the Board of the Nuclear Age Peace Foundation in Santa Barbara as well. It is a more of a lay organization, with a mission of preventing the existence of nuclear weapons.

What motivates me on a daily basis are my experiences from my childhood. I grew up in a very poor neighborhood, and as such I have always had a commitment to go back to my roots if you will, and help those who have been traditionally medically underserved. My goal is to try to prevent others from having the experiences that I had living in a very poor area of Los Angeles. I know what it is to be poor, and for that reason when I became a physician, the whole idea of wanting to serve the medically underserved has been important to me.

Serving on the National Board for Physicians for Social Responsibility, I served with Jack Geiger. He is the father of Federally Qualified Health Centers. He went to Durban, South Africa, and saw the model of care in those clinics. He gave governance of the clinics to the patients themselves. They weren't run by a healthcare organization, or university or medical school or something along those lines. He brought that model back to the United States and started clinics in Boston, where the clinics were governed by patients themselves. That is now the model of a Federally Qualified Health Center. In order for a free clinic to get federally funded, it has to have this model. The patients are the major voice in how the clinic operates. Of the governing board members, only half of them can derive income from a healthcare organization. This prevents a medical corporation or medical school from taking over the running of a community health center.

I also had the opportunity to work with Jim O'Connell who started Street Medicine. Street Medicine takes care of people where they are. His operation is also in Boston and it is pretty famous. Jim and I serve on the National Board of the Albert Schweitzer Fellowship, and it actually started at Harvard Medical School. They used to send Harvard medical students to where Albert Schweitzer had his Clinic, and about 20 years after Albert Schweitzer passed away, they wanted to entice other medical students from other medical schools to go to the Lamberene Hospital. Boston University and Tufts University went back to Harvard and said, "Why do we have to go all the way to Africa? We have the same needs in our country." So about six years ago, I started the LA Albert Schweitzer Fellowship. We tried to ask if there is any interest west of the Mississippi for any health professional student who would be willing to donate 200 hours to an agency of their choice to improve the services that the agency might provide; it can be a free clinic, community hospital, what have you. Our goal was to get health professional students engaged in trying to improve the health services that are available.

In medicine, you find that it is often similar people addressing major issues. Someone I consider to be one of the real leaders of healthcare in this country is Vivek Murthy. He was previously at Harvard's Beth Israel Deaconess Medical Center. He was active with the Albert Schweitzer Fellowship for nearly twenty years. He basically got the Surgeon General appointment because he was the founding president of what was originally Doctors for Obama, and is now Doctors for America. Someone else who was heavily involved in the Albert Schweitzer Fellowship was Former Surgeon General Regina Benjamin. She started a Catholic free clinic in the South. That same clinic was the victim of two hurricanes, and it ended up totally demolished. At basically the same time that she was rebuilding her clinic, the Catholic Church honored her with the Mother Teresa Award. Regina is now at Xavier University, where she is a professor and an endowed chair in the School of Public Health. She is still working at her clinic as a physician.

I was also one of the first volunteers for the Venice Family Clinic. I was the President of their past Board of Directors, before they became a Federally Qualified Health Center. In addition, for over 30 years, I have been volunteering at what is now called the Sabon Community Health Center and the Los Angeles Free Clinic. I also have been a volunteer for the Asian Pacific Healthcare Venture as well.

a life apart - If you have a specific emotion, you should show it, so long as it doesn't interfere with the care that you are rendering or the teaching that you are trying to do. Whether you are in a caring role or teaching role, so long as the way that we demonstrate our feelings is not counter-productive.

In terms of bonding, the physician has to understand that the patients' problems belong to the patient, and are not really the professional's problem; the role of the profession or the doctor is to help the person solve their problem. It is important to remember that the right of ownership of the problem is the patient's and not the doctor's, and to that extent the physician's role is merely to help the patient solve their own problems, rather than the physician solving the problems. I think that in so doing, the physician is going to be a lot more effective.

a lens into your life - It's interesting: every day, I find rewards in what I am doing. A lot of times you have no idea what impact your advice will play in the life of an individual. To that extent I realize that with a lot of the work that I do, I might not ever see the end result or benefit that the patients derive from interacting with me. I guess I just derive joy out of having a person reach out to me for assistance, and I do my best in trying to help the individual. And in so doing, in every interaction I have, I feel fulfillment. The feeling and mere thought that a person really in need might ultimately have a better, healthier life, as a result of the interaction they had with me, it's pretty much a gift.

I give lectures to medical students, and I give lectures to the public as well. I also see patients at a number of different family health centers. I still do a lot of volunteer work at a lot of these places. I still teach at the residency at Kaiser Permanente as well. In all the patient interactions that I still have in the various community health centers where I volunteer, I include medical students and residents. It is like I try to bring exposure for those people who would gain most from exposure to medical students and residents, so they know that the next generation will be there for them. I will say though, preventing nuclear war is my number one priority. That could be the final epidemic to afflict mankind.

John McGeehan

Cooper Medical School of Rowan University

Cooper Medical School of Rowan University is committed
to providing humanistic education in the art and science
of medicine within a scientific and scholary community in
which inclusivity, excellence in patient care, innovative
teaching, research, and service to our community are valued.

Our core values include a commitment to: diversity, personal
mentorship, professionalism, collaboration and mutual respect,
civic responsibility, patient advocacy, and life-long learning.

Dedicated July 24, 2012

John McGeehan M.D. is founding Associate Dean for Student Affairs and Admissions at the Cooper Medical School of Rowan University.

our white coat – My impression of the white coat has been amplified recently because of my ability to oversee our white coat ceremonies. What I have heard told our students is that as first year medical students, they will feel proud wearing their white coat, but not comfortable. That comfort only comes with thousands of patient experiences. The patients are the ones that will make them into doctors, not our medical school. The white coat creates an aura for individuals who hardly even know you. There are things they will share with you, that they won't even share with their own loved ones. Patients unfortunately are recently seeing the white coat in a way that isn't as therapeutic as it was before. The intense relations of patients and their doctors is fading away with the development of technology. That is the great threat to medicine much more so than the financial problems.

attending to the world - The attending physician is an individual who has chosen to teach while they care. Instead of just caring for a patient, which is important in it of itself, they have chosen to take someone under their wing, to share what they have learned over time in caring for patients. It is important that we teach students like we would teach someone how to farm. It cultivates food forever, instead of giving them food today. When a patient sees you teaching, their faith grows dramatically. Patients I have encountered over time feel better when they see me as a teacher. It cultivates a whole new element in the patient-doctor relationship.

a loving smile - That's an art that comes over time, because of the way that patients may perceive that incorrectly. There is truly a point in your career when it will just come to you. You know where that boundary is finally down, where you can be friends with a patient. When you feel comfortable as such, I think you should. Knowing when to simile, when to emphasize, when to get teary, comes with years of experience and is nothing that anybody can put in a book.Students will naturally see when and how that can occur.

a life apart - It is critical to feel sad in medicine, I look at medicine as the problem of the locked box. What I tell my students is that they will see things, hear things, and feel things that they have never felt before. If they lock those feelings in a box, and try to not bring them home, and not talk to loved ones and friends about them, it will become a habit and they will keep locking them in a black box. The problem occurs when eventually they start automatically doing it with people outside of medicine. They become this un-sharing person. Patients are clearly telling us that they don't want this type of person as their doctor. Any time you are saddened, it is ok to feel sad. I don't want any of my students to ever stop feeling.

a story - Every day I have another story. I would like to share one about a first-year student that I have now. We have something called "Week on the Wards." We have them stop classes and they get assignments all over the hospital, they experience what it is like to partake in hospital medicine. This young lady was in the intensive care unit, and saw a patient on a ventilator who was agitated. The resident team was trying to find out what was wrong with the patient who was unable to communicate. The student just choose to stay at the bedside and hold the patient's hand. She learned the next day that the patient had a full cardiac arrest. She came to me and told me what had happened. "What do you want to do?", I asked her. She replied, "I want to go to the intensive care unit and see what happened." I arranged for her to return, and she discovered that the patient had survived the cardiac arrest and had just been extubated. The gentleman looked at her, and said "you're the one who held my hand". Don't ever assume your patient doesn't know you're there and doesn't hear you. You can do magical things.

a lens - I have had an incredible life. Raised in a family who believed in me and gave me a desire to serve others, I traveled a road that allowed me to have a perfect personal and professional life. I had a private practice that became another family to me. My road led to the joy of teaching at all levels. I saw that I was not giving back as much as I had been given. I had the opportunity to play a role in creating a new medical school in the city where I had practiced for 30 years. Then came what I needed: an opportunity to help create a medical school that would be mission driven. That mission would be to change a community in need while educating tomorrow's physicians in a unique environment. My role would be to help attract those students who were driven by the same mission and give them the tools needed to serve the community that will teach them to be doctors. My current role as Associate Dean for Student Affairs and Admissions at Cooper Medical School of Rowan University in Camden, New Jersey is an opportunity beyond anything I could have imagined. We are doing something very special here. Our students will change the lives of generations to come…and they will restore a community in need. This is what I am already seeing through this lens I have been given. The picture I have chosen and attached is our school's mission set in brass on the exterior entrance to our building – and this mission has become mine.

Josh Adler

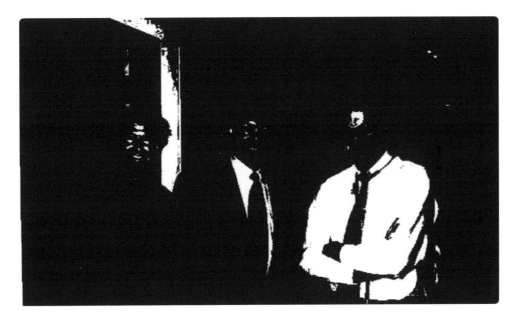

Josh Adler M.D. is Chief Medical Officer at UCSF Medical Center and UCSF Benioff Children's Hospital.

our white coat - At one level, a white coat provides patients and their families the correct identity for a physician. It ensures that there is no ambiguity. It is always important for patients to know the role and identity of the person to whom they are talking. The white coat has become expected by many patients. To show respect for patients, I wear a white coat. Yet for some people, children in particular, the white coat is a little bit scary. Thus, there are situations where it is not desirable to wear a white coat.

attending to the world - For me, being a physician gives one both the unique opportunity and unique skill set to have insight into the very intimate, perhaps most intimate, challenges that people face. Usually it is medical, or sometimes psychological, suffering. Our primary role is to try to heal and properly address this suffering. As a physician, people are willing to share such incredibly intimate details about their lives and their suffering. This comes with the expectation that you will handle that information in a compassionate way and use the information to help them. There is nothing more basic in the realm of being a citizen of the world. That is how I see the role of a medical provider.

uplifting the medically underserved - I think access to appropriate health care is a basic human right. Physicians are an important part of the delivery system, but not the only important part. It is important to emphasize that providing health care today requires a team of professionals, all of whom bring important and unique contributions to patients. The key people on the medical team include: nurses, pharmacists, physical therapists, social workers and case managers, and technicians. Moreover, whatever non-human elements are necessary, such as medications or medical tests, must be made available as well. Access to care means access to all of these professionals and services.

In my role, I have served both at UCSF and at the San Francisco Veterans Administration. In these positions, one of my primary roles is to ensure high quality care for everyone. This may mean something as simple as building a clinic closer to where people live. For example, we built clinics in much more remote areas of California, so that veterans could access care locally rather than traveling by bus to San Francisco. We attempt to provide services in a way that accounts for the specific vulnerabilities of patients. At the VA, there is fear among some veterans of the government health care system.

We find a way to create a non-threatening and therapeutic place for veterans to receive care. In the realm of my current job, we spend a lot of time thinking about racial and ethnic health disparities. Collectively we all have the responsibility to understand these disparities – and and try to eliminate them. In many cases, language is the source of health disparities. Assuring access to language interpreters for any patient who does not speak English fluently, and even those who do speak English fluently but prefer to converse in their native language, is a key responsibility of health care leaders and can reduce health disparities. Cultural differences are important to consider as well. For example, when engaging in discussions about death, health care professionals need to consider to consider a patient and family's culture. Different approaches are required to properly address the needs of patients from different cultures. In order to reduce health disparities, leaders must constantly ask, "Are we doing this the right way?" It will lead your organization on a path towards combating and eliminating disparities.

a loving smile - I absolutely think it is appropriate for physicians to bond with patients, and I think it is a part of the mutual healing process that goes on when patients have more than just a transactional relationship with a physician. That is not to say though that a physician will find it easy to emotionally bond with every patient that comes through the door. I think that it is unrealistic to expect that an emotional bond should occur between a physician and every single patient. If it does occur, it is generally therapeutic for both patients and physicians. It is certainly okay to hug a patient or hold a patient's hand when they are crying or may have just received some bad news. For many patients such a gesture can be therapeutic and is part of what caregiving means as a physician. The same goes for family members, especially when a physician knows a family for a long time. I think it is helpful for patients to see that a physician is also moved by good or bad news. There are nonetheless limits to this type of emotional bonding. Physicians must be able to remain objective when it comes to advising patients, medical decision making, and using scientific evidence in the practice of medicine. This objectivity is at the core of the professional relationship between patients and physicians.

a story - When I was working at the Veterans Administration Hospital, we received a call from General Colin Powell, then Chairman of the Joint Chiefs of Staff. He asked to come by that morning to meet with veterans in the hospital. He asked that there not be any press or media involved. He arrived at 7 a.m. and asked me to accompany him to introduce him to our patients and vice versa. That day, there were roughly 220 veterans in the hospital and he met with every single one. He introduced himself, thanked them for their service, and then saw the next person. I still remember that day as one of the most therapeutic days I have ever spent in a hospital both for our patients and for all of us who worked there. Every one of those Veterans was just on "cloud nine." It was a great thing to be a part of. Though it had very little to do with the practice of medicine, it was a wonderful lesson in leadership. Attached is a picture of me with General Powell and one of my mentors, Dr. Lawrence Tierney. For all of us, including patients, physicians, nurses, and hospital chiefs of staff, it was one of the greatest days in the history of the San Francisco VA. General Powell demonstrated real compassion and appreciation for his team (the U.S. military) in a humble and transparent way.

Laurie Glimcher

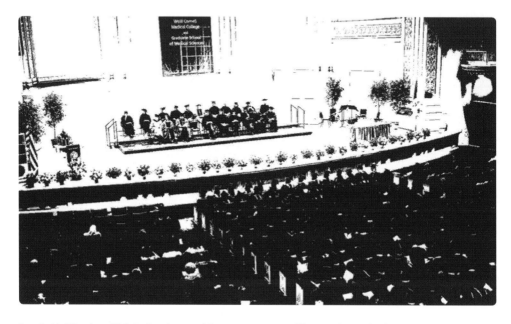

Laurie H. Glimcher, M.D. is Stephen and Suzanne Weiss Dean at Weill Cornell Medical College.

attending to the world - I have spent the majority of my career doing biomedical research in immunology, and my goal as Dean is to facilitate the translation of discoveries at the bench into new therapies for patients.

It's important that we go from bench to bedside- and equally important that we go from bedside back to bench. Most discoveries are inspired by insights at the bedside by observant clinicians.

Michael Drake

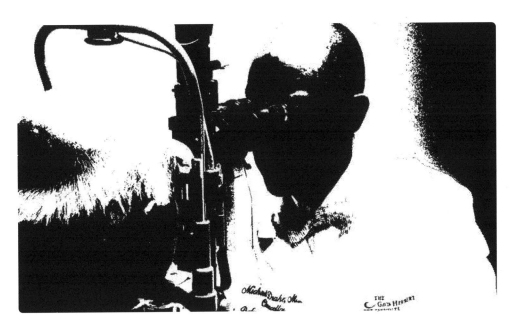

Michael V. Drake, M.D. is former Chancellor of the University of California, Irvine, and Professor of Opthalmology at the University of California, Irvine School of Medicine; and currently serves as President of The Ohio State University.

our white coat - The most special part of the doctor-patient relationship is how it's built on the bond of trust. The patient, in sharing his scariest secrets, is as vulnerable as he has ever been. The doctor must honor that trust by applying her years of training and experience to address the patient's fears. It is a collaboration with the common goal of healing.

attending to the world - Teaching is sharing information so that the student has something she did not have before. The hallmark of the profession is this transfer to the next generation. It has an exponential effect. You serve the learner, the learner's patients, the learner's students, and yourself.

a loving smile - The doctor-patient relationship begins with and is defined by the person-to-person relationship. Truly loving people is a characteristic of a good physician.

a life apart - Empathy and compassion make us human. They add texture, richness, and satisfaction to our relationships with patients. When things are not going well for a patient, sadness becomes a factor, but we must move forward in our sadness to continue helping.

a story - Years ago I had a student who came to medicine from a career as a marine biologist. When working alone in the Gulf of Mexico, he spent hours helping a small beached whale return to the sea. When he boated back to the mainland that evening, he decided he wanted to experience that feeling again.

Michelle Forcier

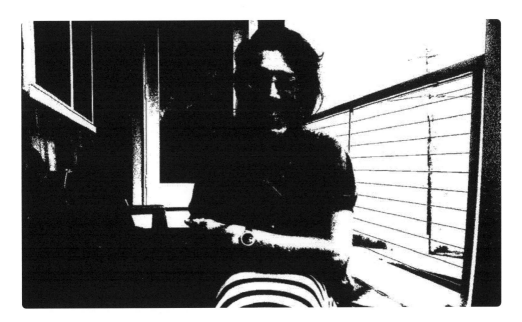

Michelle Forcier M.D. is Assistant Dean for Medical Education and Associate Professor of Pediatrics at the Alpert Medical School of Brown University. She is considered by many to be the nation's expert on transgender medicine.

our white coat - The first thing for me is that I don't use the white coat for working with children. The white coat becomes somewhat of a barrier and a visible symbol of power. I tend to dress informally and casually ; I think it may make me more approachable. I tend to reject the white coat ostensibly because it sets up a hierarchy of power. What we can do instead of hiding behind the white coat is offer ourselves in the visit to be present, to be of service. One of the first phrases that can build patient centered care is "what can I do for you? What brings you here to our clinic? How might I be most helpful." It is the same thing you would say if you worked in a restaurant serving coffee or if you were at a store trying to help someone find an item. I reject the white coat to create a level playing ground with the children I serve. This approach lends me the chance to connect person-to-person and makes the relationship all about service.

attending to the world - Medicine is full of these double entendres. For instance, you have your "practice", your practice being your clinical services that you can offer, what you know, what you might recommend. Every day we realign and revisit and retry the of science of medicine. We continue to practice what we know and sometimes what we don't know but think it may be useful to the patient… We "practice" growing our art, knowledge, skills of medicine. The same thing for the attending physician who should be supervising the resident and medical students and supervising the big picture for the patient. Attending as part of our practice means paying attention and validating the details of the big picture, making sure that everything gets done the way that it is supposed to get done, attending to the patient at his or her core, attending to the patient's needs, to the patient's body language, the patient's anxiety and concerns, attending to the patient's family and how that interplays with the past. Giving good care requires paying attention and are responsive to your patient needs.

a loving smile - It is appropriate to bond with patients; each day; bonding can mean different things. Being attentive and responsive, allows you to learn what the patient wants and needs and the different ways to bond and support. Some patients respond more to warmth and empathy. Other patients don't really want that from you. When they are clear that they want distance, you can embody a calm, cool, collected physician presence. The bond should be there, as a professional the physician needs to implicitly read into what the patient is asking for that visit or that day, in that particular time, in that person's life. The physician should respond with emotion and interpersonal presence. If you miss the importance of intimacy, you will miss important medical and cultural information. You need to do everything you can to understand how a patient might want to meet you in the middle.

I have hugged patients and gotten teary-eyed in front of my patients. In the end, I hope it helped me communicate something of value. As long as you are truly doing that inner values clarification, you can sometimes move beyond traditional boundaries and offer something of use to a patient.

I often ask myself, "was this sharing of emotion just for me or the patient?" If it is for the patient, then I think it is definitely ok.

a life apart - Unfortunately, in medicine, while you see some fantastic and amazing, wonderful moments in peoples' lives, you sometimes see the worst of what happens to people and also by people. Having a minute to really rejoice and celebrate or be sad, mourn and even be angry for your patients is important. Feelings shouldn't interfere with your ability to provide patient-centered care, yet not feeling would be a barrier to paying attention and the ability to intellectually and emotionally respond. I often feel sad when a patient can't afford the basics, when a patient's loved one isn't seeing or listening to them, when they can't receive the care that they need. Being present might mean supporting them in making the decisions that they, and not you, need to make. When I feel sad, when life is unfair, when the luck of the draw is wrong, when good people are hurt or suffering, sometimes the only thing I can offer a patient is "being present" and being supportive. For the patients who transform gender or have a non-conforming status, I feel particularly bad when they have to go through the headache and extra work and hassle our system creates. Feeling a want and a wish for people to be happy and safe and well is emotional, but is also doctoring. I'm not sure I have it yet, but I know I'm reaching for it.

a story - I think if you are here for the right reasons, you hear some life changing, amazing stories. I work with a lot of powerful and amazing kids. Together, they are doing some transformative work together. My most powerful patient is the patient that I feel like was my biggest mistake. The patient that I am thinking about came to me in the 1990's before there was a lot of internet and electronic information readily available. He was a really nice young man. He was biologically a female but identified as a male. He was very clear on this. He had been expressing as masculine for a while. This young person who clearly wanted to transition to male gender and sought my help. He had a period which he hated, and we figured one of the things we

could do was stop his period. We thought he wanted to do more in the way of hormones and transition. In the 1990's, there was not a lot out about and for transgender kids. We sent him to a pediatric endocrinologist. They said, "We can't do anything until this kid is of legal age." It just felt so wrong.

We didn't know what else we could do. We didn't offer him what he really needed. I learned that sometimes doing nothing is harm. Not allowing or helping a transgender patient to move forward to their asserted gender is harm, not finding a patient a way to transform in a safe, healthy and supported way is harm. I talk about this a lot at conferences and with my patients today. Most of these kids, most transgender pubertal youth in non-conforming status, are not going to change their minds. Parents are often very afraid they are going to make the wrong consent decision and make the wrong choice for their child's future. They ask me, how can this 14 year old know he doesn't want a period? Or children some day? We know that when we don't pay attention to the adolescent, the outcomes are much poorer in the long term. If we listen and say we hear you and this is what we can do to help you, we can facilitate more positive outcomes. Of course you don't want to make a mistake as a physician, so it is scary at times. You don't want to do something that seems so extravagant. Yet to quote one of my kids, "it really is powerful seeing the alternative of not living in your true identity can be so bad. This pushes you forward." Not doing something can be the most harmful thing we do; not listening, not taking a youth seriously, and not trying to find a way can be dangerous. I don't know what happened to this one kid. I know that when I was there, he was in and out of care. As time went on I don't know.

I was at one of the oldest transgender meetings in the US talking to all these wonderful 50, 60, 70 year old transgender individuals who were clearly looking back. Many of them said, if I had care earlier, I wouldn't have had to live my entire life in the closet. I would have been able to identify as female, have a quality of life and job, and date or have a family, and be able to secure housing. So I think that from talking with my older trans patients, I know that if they had more available earlier, they would have been able to go a lot farther in embracing their true feminine or masculine self more naturally over the course of their lifetime.

a lens into your life - I often walk into a room where there is a very anxious youth and patient. Because they may have had some bad experiences in the past, we introduce ourselves first. We ask if they want to tell us a little bit about what brings them there and what would make for a really good visit. We talk about our paradigm of gender and human development. This introduction attempts to normalize diversity in gender, de-stigmatize when kids and adults are gender variant, and open the door to a very open conversation. I try to set up our visit based on transparency and modifying our paradigm to the patient's needs. We are judged in so many different ways that so many gender non-conforming youth are very excited to have this conversation. Some feel that having this conversation is taboo, or that the details are so sensitive that we try and take a background history first so we get to know the whole person. When we open the door to a patient's room, we say who we are and ask if there is anything we can do to make them feel more safe and comfortable. We have these wonderful conversations about their lives and experiences, and gender identity, and hopes and dreams for who they will be in terms of their male or female gender. Making the welcome and safety aspect needs to be explicit, so that they know this can be a place where they will feel safe and welcome always. At the end, we discuss a menu of options for care; and from truly a sort of service perspective, I ask "How did the visit go for you?" I have them rate it on a scale where 1 is incredibly sucky and 8-9 where this is really good. I tell patients I am curious to know what made the visit valuable for them; or what we need to change since it did not work so well. It is all about the experience, the relationship and the patient at the center. Whether the patient is a kid or an adult, we really encourage their feedback. We want to make sure that we open the door in both directions. In earlier time, transgender individuals may have had to prove their asserted gender - patients don't have to prove anything to us. We listen and learn from them.

Millard Collins

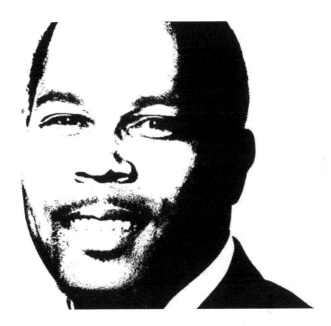

Millard Collins M.D. is Associate Dean for Student and Academic Affairs at Meharry Medical College.

our white coat - I guess my answer will address both of these. The white coat is kind of a blessing and a curse. Starting with the bad, for example, people refer to "white coat hypertension". I think in this way it can be seen as a barrier. Lots of patients from underserved communities can be very intimidated by the white coat. They feel that you may judge them, because they may not be very health literate or have routine care.

Many of these people come from poor, disadvantaged backgrounds and can be sensitive to redirection or basic explanations. I tell my students, "Sit down, and look at them face to face. It will make you a little more effective as a provider."

The power of the white coat can be overwhelming. At the same time, it is a part of the uniform. It can give some people hope; hope that you may be able to offer them help that will make them more comfortable when they are scared and unsure about their circumstances. In terms of being able to facilitate healing both ways, the true patient provider, provides an experience where patients can trust you for the right reasons; because they know you care about them. The white coat gives you the highest order of respect and responsibility. By getting to know patients as people, they will open up a little bit more; we can only help our patients as much as they are honest with us and willing to provide us with accurate information. Many people just have past anxiety, and once they see who you actually are, I think they accept that there is a person behind the white coat.

attending to the world - I like analogies. I played sports all my life; I was pretty good at some things. Much like sports stars and actors, and other different fields, it takes a person with the necessary skills, knowledge, and talent to be a physician. With such skills, I cannot stress compassion and empathy enough - that you really care about helping people. If you take the Hippocratic Oath seriously, you can make a difference in people's lives every day. It is a duty, and it's an awesome duty. If you are bringing someone into this world, or helping someone transition into the next life, it's an awesome responsibility and a privilege to stand with people who are facing the ultimate suffering and sometimes, who have been forgotten. We meet our clients where they are. Attending to the world is the duty of every physician. Not everyone can do it, but for those with the skills and compassion, it is the biggest honor one can have.

uplifting the medically underserved - Sometimes we look at the world as "haves and have nots". Even in America, it is a shame that people are still underserved. It is one of the biggest travesties. Here at Meharry, we believe in the "Worship of God Through Service to Mankind". As a physician-educator, it feels truly remarkable when you are able to teach someone to truly care about mankind. It's not just about access, it's about care. Each physician has a tremendous role in shaping the doctors of tomorrow. We need to teach people to walk the walk and not just talk the talk. We need people with a sense of mission, who are selfless.

One time I was in a code with a 25 year old patient. One of the physician's quick wit caused an eruption of laughter. I knew his brother was behind the curtain. I stepped out and he was devastated. "There are people laughing while my brother is dying". I explained that if these people truly put themselves in the moment, they would be unable to function and do their job. While this made him feel better, such behavior is not acceptable in medicine. We can't make our patients or their families uncomfortable to fit into our roles. We need to find the courage inside to fit into our roles.

a loving smile - I think medicine is all about our repertoire and bonding- building relationships. I had a chief resident who taught me the effect of looking at someone with a big smile, regardless of what is going on in our personal lives or theirs. Satisfaction in care and satisfaction in life all starts with a smile. I tell my medical students, instead of focusing on the adversities, focus on three things that will make you happy. There are many things you simply can't cure; you can't cure someone of an incurable disease, but if you teach that patient how to smile, you can lead them on the road to happiness.

a life apart - I have friends who come to see me as their physician. "How can you treat a friend if you cannot separate the two?" I am often asked. It is something that you can become accustomed to through training and experience. I think a main goal needs to be being able to stay in the moment. If we are able to focus on the moment and the task at hand, we can take care of medical needs while really caring about people.

a story - This is one I share with my students. We serve at the County Hospital, and there are lots of indigent patients who come in in the winter- hungry, cold, sick, disheveled. It is not a place to turn, because the hospital can't provide everything they need. I walk in the room. I'm a greeter; I shake this patient's hand. As I'm talking to the group, one of the students motioned that the guy was tearful. He said, "I'm fine, I feel extremely blessed right now, because being with you is making me feel better. You are the first person to walk up to me and look me in the face and just shake my hand in many years." He was dirty, disheveled. I just remember him. He had a rough break in life, but he was someone's son and born just like you and

me. If you just realize the positive effect of putting your hand out and on someone's shoulder, you can make a world of a difference.

I tell my students, next time you are at a stop light and it is cold, just look around and look at the homeless people on benches. Look at the world around them. We tend to forget about them. Our society has forgotten about them. Try to treat them like human beings, try to just give them some of the respect they deserve.

a lens into your life - I have the best job in the world. I'm a family physician. An ideal day for me would be one where I get to care for elderly patients at the nursing home in the morning - often people from low-income backgrounds who have been forgotten by society. Then I would head back to the clinic. I'd do a well child visit for a six-month-old getting immunizations. Then I'd advise someone on pregnancy, and maybe help with a surgical intervention. Sometimes they don't want to receive care, and I remind them that their father would really want for them to have a life. It's always awesome when I can give someone insight that helps them to feel better about the decisions that they are making. On the same day, I'll counsel someone at the end of life, and then go meet with parents who are excited and anxious about bringing life into this world. People share with me experiences that are meaningful, and unique, and important in their lives. When I treat each patient, I approach it as if they are the most important person in the world. I give them my full heart and attention. When I think about the impact I want to make, I start to think about my father. While he was not a physician, he was an incredibly caring man. Since we have the same name, it is my dream to have his name on a building one day. I try to represent everything he lived for, so it would be the ultimate gift I could honor him with. I tell people I think that I have the best job in the world. I am so grateful I got to be a physician.

Pascal Goldschmidt

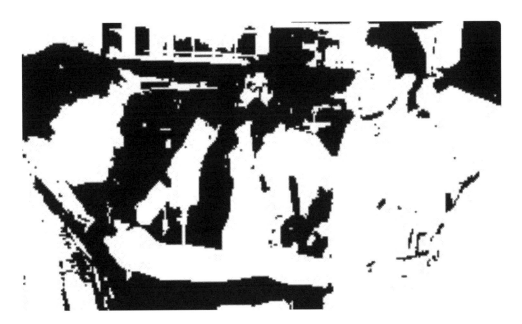

Pascal Goldschmidt M.D. is Dean of the University of Miami Miller School of Medicine, and Chief Medical Officer of the University of Miami Health System.

our white coat - I think that fundamentally, patients participate substantially in their healing. I was just listening to Magic Johnson speak, and the way he talks about his journey through HIV/AIDS is remarkable. One thing that is very clear is that what he has said about the importance of taking medications for his condition saved countless lives in the U.S. and around the world.

He explained beautifully that his mindset was that he wanted to live for his family, his children and grandchildren. Yes, good evidence-based medicine played a pivotal role in improving the drugs that became available to treat HIV/AIDS, but Magic Johnson was critical to changing the course of the epidemic. I think it is true for me, as a cardiologist, that when patients come in with an acute heart attack, they look for support and comfort. You can improve their condition, blood pressure, heart rate and even oxygenation substantially just by listening and telling them that they came to the right team that will do everything possible to get them better. And then, of course, one needs to apply the cutting-edge technologies of modern medicine.

attending to the world - I am the Dean of the Miller School of Medicine, and there is an extraordinary contract between each medical school and society. We educate and evaluate future physicians, and when we provide them with a degree, we are signing a contract with society. We are saying that these individuals are capable of dealing with the highest level of trust, which is to put your health in their hands. We are telling society that these individuals will be competent and responsible partners in managing your health. We are telling society that these individuals have the proper ethics and accountability to deal with such responsibility in an effective and ethical way.

uplifting the medically underserved - How do you make sure that the uninsured will have access at least once a year to preventive care? Of all that we can do for a patient, prevention is probably the most fundamental and effective aspect of care, but for many reasons it is actually not easy for uninsured patients to access preventive care. Our Miller medical students organize nine health fairs each year, with the generous support of our faculty. The last health fair was a few blocks away from my office in Little Haiti, and we saw more than 350 people. These individuals had an average contact of 55 minutes with a care provider -- more than they could expect from an encounter with a primary

care provider. They each received a full review of their health condition with an interview, assessment of vital signs, and a full physical including an eye exam and a prostate or gynecological exam by our physician specialists. It is a huge commitment, but it is a very important one that we owe to our community. We take it very seriously; it involved hundreds of volunteer faculty, students and staff, and it is critical to guarantee that these patients will have that one disease prevention opportunity each year.

For those individuals we do not have the opportunity to evaluate, because we are often overwhelmed by the pent-up demand, we refer them to the free clinics where we work frequently and where they will be able to access quality care. In addition to these community services, about 60 percent of our faculty physicians work at the safety net hospital, Jackson Memorial Hospital, where the poorest and the richest receive the same level of care. It is an important commitment for our medical school; we see it as of critical importance in our mission to improve the health of this community. You can see the impact on the region, and we wish we could do more. The patients who rely on Jackson as a safety net hospital are typically individuals who would have no access to primary or other care. Hopefully, some will be able to access insurance under the Affordable Care Act, yet some of them are not legal immigrants and do not have the relevant paperwork. As a consequence, even with this new legislation, they will not be covered. They are usually new immigrants, people who came to work low-paying jobs in the United States. They frequently are the individuals who take advantage of our health fairs and free clinic services. The name of our student-run program is DOCS (Department of Community Service); it is overseen by board-certified Miller School physicians. We are in the process of producing documentaries to encourage students at other institutions to do the same, and we provide guidance to other medical schools in starting similar community service initiatives.

a loving smile - I think that you always bond with your patients. The intensity of the bond is an issue of time, but even if you see a patient for several minutes you can still develop some bond. Some patients are more apt to create bonds than others. If you are a physician who is more prone to bonding, you will certainly do it effectively with most of your patients. There are limits to that too. You have to define some boundaries so that your life is not completely depleted of contact with your own family. Your own physical activity is an important part of your ability to cope with a demanding professional life; it will keep you in good health and give you a level of energy you can share.

a life apart - Maybe one of the reasons to choose a certain medical discipline over others is that we have different levels of resistance to difficult situations. For example, I have a passion for oncology, but I do not think I could emotionally deal with being a pediatric oncologist. I recognize the critical importance of that

discipline, which is absolutely essential for our children. However, I do not think that I could actually practice it every day. It does not mean that there is something wrong with me; we have the toolbox that we have. Some people are more capable of putting emotional barriers between their sensitivity and their daily work life. Yet if I find myself in an emotionally challenging situation, it will never prevent me from being extremely efficient at what I do. However, as a day-to-day activity, it would probably push me to the limits of what I can handle.

a story - I talk to medical students the first day they come to the school year after year. I can tell you that what excites them is when you tell them a story. After the earthquake in Haiti in 2010, doctors, nurses and staff of the Miller School went to Port-Au-Prince within 24 hours and built a 250-bed field hospital where we cared for Haitians for several months until other structures again became available. We helped the physicians' transition from the field hospital to a more permanent trauma and general hospital. Dr. Barth Green, our chair of neurosurgery, has been overseeing this effort in the past few years since the earthquake. These are the kinds of stories that motivate students and make them realize that everything is possible in medicine. What you put in is what you are going to get out. If you want to serve your fellow humans there is no better job. At the end of the day, we have to fulfill the goal that we had the first day of medical school. Some people are more gifted than others, but we can all fulfill the goal of service. We really have to sit down from time to time as physicians and ask ourselves, "Am I still keeping up the commitment that I dedicated my life to – which is to help our fellow humans through medicine?"

a lens into your life - In action with a few colleagues from Miller School of Medicine/ UHealth, Port Au Prince, Haiti, January 15, 2010. The boy on the stretcher had a bad case of renal failure due to rhabdomyolysis. Barth Green, Neurosurgery Chair at UM, was leading the effort. Most of our employees did participate, either on site, or at home covering for their colleagues.

Paul Roth

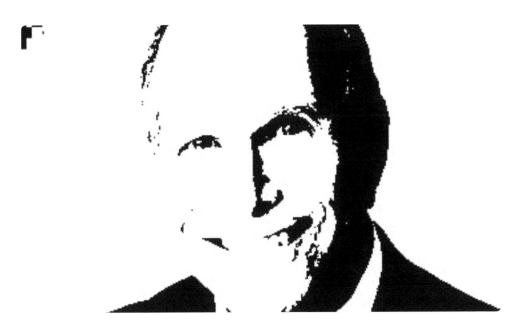

Paul Roth M.D. trained in emergency medicine and currently serves as Chancellor of the University of New Mexico School of Medicine.

our white coat - The white coat symbolizes a physician's dedication to serving others and to the humanistic values of medicine. This commitment is celebrated each year in our white coat ceremony for new medical students whereat they recite the Oath of Geneva for the first time and hear stories of its real-life significance from other more senior students and faculty. This experience continues to be as moving for me as it is for our students and their families. It evokes the values of the profession we have all chosen--combining a balanced approach to patient care based on scientific knowledge with a compassionate wisdom for the whole patient's well-being.

attending to the world - Service to others is the foundation for everything we do as physicians. This entails placing the patient's interests and well-being above our own. This is true whether you are at the bedside with an individual patient or in the executive suite addressing the health needs of populations.

uplifting the medically underserved - You probably could speak to lots of physicians from various specialties; the more uniform answer from doctors in the ED is that there is no place where disparities are more obvious than the emergency department. Many years ago, patients could be turned away if they didn't have money or insurance, now

there are laws that require them to treat you, no one can be turned away. I guess emergency departments are really the front door of the hospital. They are used frequently by people who have no other place to go. Helping people who are in your beds and when your beds are full, even in the waiting room. I often view my "office" as the place where I get to take care of everyone, regardless of whether anyone else chooses to treat them. Emergency medicine is the field where we recognize that we are a final, common pathway for everyone to be seen. It can be a challenge, yet I think it is a blessing that you get to be there for these patients.

a loving smile - Truly "being there" with a patient is extraordinarily powerful. Making eye contact, being attentive to what your patient is communicating to you and responding compassionately can make a huge difference.

a life apart - Striking the right balance between work and family is paramount. We must understand that we all serve as role models for family and community, and therefore, should live by the healthy behaviors we expect from our patients.

a story - I was attending in the ER several years ago when the front clerk ran up quite distressed saying that she thought a person was dead in our lobby! I discovered an elderly woman limp and slumped over in her chair and found her to be pulseless and without respirations. Shocked, my first impulse was to pick the patient up in my arms and run with her into our resuscitation room, yelling for help along the way. We began advanced cardiac life support, and to make a long story short, she left the hospital two weeks later. About a month afterward, she came to the ER with tears in her eyes, carrying a tray of home-baked cookies to thank me for what we all had done. I smile each time I recall this very dramatic encounter. It only takes an occasional success, that one moment when one knows that all the years of training, study, and dedication can save a life. That moment keeps my spirits high and provides constant motivation to do all in my power to better the lives of those we serve.

a lens into your life - Now that I spend most of my time as a physician executive, I try to maintain the mindset described above, whether developing high-level strategies or solving daily problems. I believe this leads to better, more meaningful outcomes.

Philip Pizzo

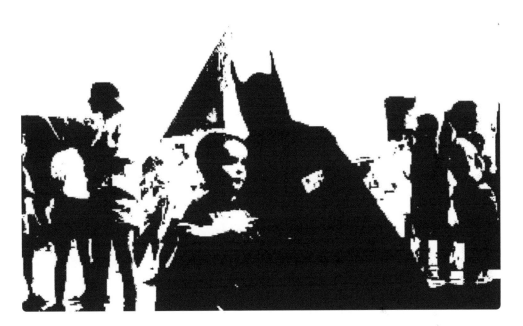

Philip Pizzo M.D. is Former Dean and the David and Susan Heckerman Professor of Pediatrics and of Microbiology and Immunology, at Stanford University School of Medicine

our white coat - By way of context, I need to tell you a little bit about the areas of medicine that I have been involved with over the years. In broad terms, pediatrics and more specifically, pediatric oncology and pediatric infectious diseases. I have spent a lot of time working with both children and their families, in particular those who have complex medical conditions,

from children with cancer, those with complicated infectious disorders and children with HIV infections. Importantly, pediatricians tend to be more focused on how to meet the needs of both the patient and his or her family. The patient-doctor relationship depends on the desires of the family as well as whether the patient is a child or adolescent. A different kind of relationship is required depending upon age. The model of pediatric care is by definition more family centric, and I believe is also a good model for medicine in general.

In general, pediatrics tends to be very cognizant of the dynamics of disease. Pediatric diseases never just impact a single person, they usually impact an entire family and community, and require a special caring touch from the physician. Speaking broadly, when discussing complex disorders, it always requires collaboration with the family in a proactive way. There is a need to be sympathetic and compassionate in a manner that simultaneously allows one to facilitate a fact-based discussion on what the problems are and what the potential interventions might be. At the same time, it is important that the patient, the child, understands the intervention as well as possible. This requires time and patience. Shared understanding is a core necessity of the relationship one has to have with his or her patients. I have been a part of medicine for many years, and it seems there is can never be enough listening or hearing patients' concerns and showing genuine interest on the part of the physician. This is something that we all need to work on. More often there is too much direction and talking on the part of the caregivers without contextualizing it into the unique social setting of the individual. Patients come from very different cultural and social backgrounds; and our message must be modified according to that. We must collaborate in a way that responds to the unique background and questions raised by each patient and his or her family.

attending to the world - Physicians should approach clinical interactions from a patient- and family-centric perspective. And they need to be aware that the words they use and the way they deliver their message has an enormous impact the family. Illness is not just a physical state; it is a biopsychosocial issue. It is a biological problem at the intersection of society, and behavioral issues can alter the disease. The solution is shaped by what the individual is willing to do with the information received from the physician and other care providers.

uplifting the medically underserved - This is an enormously important issue. We live in a very sad state of reality, where healthcare is not viewed as a human right in the US. Over the greater part of the 20th century, the United States still has not developed an organized healthcare system as other developed countries have done. We have a model that evolved over decades that went from patient centrality to doctor and medical system centrality. Medicine has lost its focus on providing better health for individuals, in particular those who are uninsured or underserved. As a result many of these people's healthcare comes from visits to the emergency room. It is a pretty disgraceful state of affairs. Delivery and reform and advanced prevention measures are things that I am a big advocate for. The single payer system would provide a much better answer for both healthcare and for the finances that come in concert with it. We can achieve equity in many different ways, and using many different models. Our model needs to be re-calibrated so that it focuses on what patients need and how to provide them health in a proactive way, as opposed to the current model, in which institutions construct their healthcare delivery systems so that they operate with a profit-margin perspective.

a loving smile - It is enormously important to form a human bond with every patient that one sees. One of the dangers of modern medicine is that there has been an increasing separation of the physician as a humanistic care provider, as we see that technology permits us to diagnose and interact with patients from a distance in ways that almost remove the need for the human touch. What patients tell us they want and feel is that very human connection. They want an individual who is a care provider to sit down and to connect with them, and reach out, and make a human connection. Whether a patient or a family member, each person wants to share some witnessing of the fact that they are part of a dynamic process. Your first question to me began with the "white coat", it is a symbol of medicine and yet it is also a symbol of distance as well. Even if someone is wearing a white coat, one needs to convey that as a provider you are there as a person too. The other instrument that some might say we don't really need any longer is the stethoscope, yet I believe it is an important symbol because it connects one directly to the patient. I think that those connections at the heart of your questions, direct physical contact, doing the exam in a compassionate and caring way, listening at a level that shows the patient you are part of the dialogue and not towering over them. I would say that these are the most important attributes of being an effective physician.

a life apart - As someone who has been involved with children facing life-threatening disease, two aspects of care have come to be particularly important to me. I have learned over many decades of time, that it is important to find ways for compartmentalizing the process of care delivery. Even though part of my life has been dealing with human tragedy and disease, it is important for the physician to find a way to be able to shield one's personal life from it so that you can continue being effective. At the same time, in each interaction with a patient and his or her family, it is important from my point of view to enter each relationship in a deeply sincere manner. The times in my life when I have sat down with a child or family who was facing a life-challenging situation, I have always felt a tremendous sense of burden on behalf of the child and family, and they often shared that sense of evocative emotion with me. It has always been important to me to listen in a deeply humanistic and caring way. I think it is appropriate to allow trainees to be part of the listening process and experience that evocative emotion. If one completely compartmentalizes their feelings, it lessens their effectiveness as a humanistic, caring person in medicine. It is all about balance, because if you bring those emotions with you outside of the patient setting, it impacts negatively on a physician's ability to lead a healthy normal life himself. However, if you really connect with a patient it is of course okay to tip the balance a little bit. It is really about knowing who you are.

a story - I'm going to give an example of a situation that changed my life; it didn't happen as a first year medical student, it happened during my training. From my research to my clinical work, I have strived to make an impact. I was treating a young boy who had aplastic anemia. He was ten years of age, and was placed by a group of well meaning and caring physicians and providers into a protected environment, a sterile setting that meant his only contact with people were with providers in sterile garb. The goal was to prevent him from getting a serious infection when his blood counts were very low. Over the course of seven years of treatment, I was his physician for most of the time, and he demonstrated an incredible degree of human resilience to his life journey. This youngster continued to reach out and grow, and develop human relationships. It underscored the basic drive to be well even when facing catastrophic disease. This is an example of a dramatic situation, but there are many others that have occurred in my life where individuals who were facing a horrendous disease seemed to find ways to surmount it. In essence, this youngster's actions forced me to reach a higher level of responsibility, to address problems when the information is unknown for all the potential solutions. We had to find ways of improving the care environment to help him overcome the the limitations he faced everyday. Being able to do this in someone else's life

is why many of us went into medicine, in order to be care providers, to be inventors and discoverers, to be individuals who heal and learn to interact with the human condition in ways that allow people to continue to do well with whatever life and time they have.

a lens into your life - I have had a great opportunity to lead many lives as a physician-leader, from being a direct care provider, to a leader of research and clinical team, to being an institutional leader of a large children's hospital and medical school. To me, being a physician means bringing knowledge forward and sharing it well in order to overcome obstacles whether in the administrative bodies of life or societal struggles. When one looks closely at the course of a physician's life, in many ways every day is filled with new opportunities for both learning and for healing. I often tell our medical students here at Stanford that after decades of being a leader in medicine and in science I have never felt that I was coming to work. I've never had a job in a traditional sense of the word. It is always a feeling of mission and wonderment. The things we can do, learn, and help a student learn. Learning from someone else, overcoming a block or obstacle, finding oneself or a peer as a route to new discovery, all of those things are wrapped in a life in medicine and science. Those experiences inspire me to this day, and make me want to continue to do things that resonate well on behalf of life and society.

Robert Grant

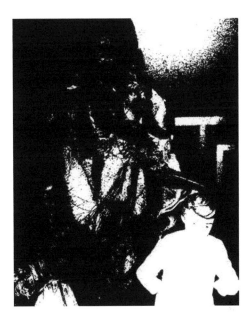

Robert Grant M.D. is a Professor of Virology at UCSF, Director of the Gladstone Institute, and on *Time Magazine*'s 2012 list of 100 Most Influential People in the World: #20, Most Influential Physician.

our white coat - Any human interaction involves two sides at least. In many cases, there are three or four sides. There are entire communities that are involved with each patient's life. Any human interaction that person has, whether with a parent, a grandparent, or a child, is a part of that community. The white coat is a part of

that community. I think that there are times when the white coat has uses, and others when it does not. When people who are suffering from disease see the white coat, they are sometimes reassured to see a physician who is dressed in a way that seems clean and organized. But there are other times when that just gets in the way, when the coat becomes a barrier. I sometimes practice in the ICU, which is a setting where some people appreciate white coats, because there is so much going on in those environments. There is so much uncertainty and a lot of bacteria, and having a white coat just makes it feel cleaner. In the outpatient setting, I would never wear a white coat. People and providers should meet each other as peers as best they can. We shouldn't pretend that our world and life are clean of illness. We have to go halfway to get to the patient.

attending to the world - I have always enjoyed the word attending. It is really the right word. Much of what we do in medicine is to attend – to just be present with suffering, to be present with illness, to be present with questions, to be present to offer suggestions, and to be present to comfort. Being an attending is providing a service to the patient, to the world, and in many situations the only service we can provide is to be present in every way possible. Interacting and responding are our responsibilities as clinicians, but responding often means just being present.

uplifting the medically underserved - Helping each other heal including treatment, diagnosis, and palliative care are fundamental human rights. They are more than that – they are fundamental human activities and some of the most marvelous things we do for each other as human beings. Cooking for each other, feeding each other, touching each other, talking with each other, just spending time with each other, these are amazingly important human interactions. They make our lives special. They make our lives vibrant, and healing is one of those activities that is quintessentially human. We should participate in that frequently. I do be-

lieve it is a right, just as people have the right to education. The right to health care services is something that our society owes to every single person. I think that people get that. If you ever hear a story about someone who becomes sick, it is never acceptable that they could not find a doctor. There are people who are sick and who do not have access, and when any one of us hear about one those situations, we feel compelled to do something about it. The truth is that society failed that person. People as a whole recognize that it is a human right. Whether they are willing to acknowledge it and do anything arises from person to person. It is impossible for me to stand by when people are suffering from disease. I am just compelled to do something about it when I see it.

a loving smile - I think that the health care provider and the patient always have a certain amount of bonding that occurs. Both people are vulnerable, both people are struggling, although struggling with different aspects of the challenge. The patient is dealing with the condition, and the provider is suffering to find the most effective way to palliate, diagnose, and cure. Everyone there is struggling, and they are struggling together. That is a form of bonding. It is important to have boundaries too. The interaction is mainly focused on the patient's need to receive a diagnosis and some level of comfort. That should govern the relationship, and bonding in other ways is almost always going to be confusing to one or the other party. I think that the doctor and patient relationship is one that is very special and should be respected. It is not like other relationships.

a life apart - I think it is always okay to feel sad, and I think we need to acknowledge our own feelings. Being present and attending to other people's suffering and their disease means being present for ourselves as well. When we feel sad, we absolutely have to feel sad. I think it is always okay to feel sad if the situation calls for it. Sometimes there's nothing else you can do than to actually commiserate with people. Our feeling sad should not ever mean that we stop thinking of a better solution, stop thinking of treatments, stop thinking of alternative diagnosis. Feelings of sadness that are genuine never make us stop thinking. It takes time to develop a meaningful relationship with each patient, and the provider must ensure that they care for him or herself in the process. It is also always important for physicians to have pleasures in their lives that allow themselves to heal as well.

a story - The story of my life as a medical student was when I was a first year at UCSF and a public health student at UC Berkeley. I was looking for a job because I needed one to help pay expenses, and I wanted to work as a research associate. One of the faculty said, you should go to Dr. Winklestein, a Professor of Epidemiology, because he just got a big grant to study a new disease, and there was a lot of work to be done. He said, in fact, we are studying an emerging disease that is killing people, and we don't really understand what it is. It turned out

to be Acquired Immune Deficiency Syndrome. As soon as I started working in that field, I felt completely fulfilled as a medical student. I had gone to medical school wanting to be a practicing physician and not thinking of being a researcher at all. When faced with the frightening mysteries of AIDS, I wanted nothing other to study than finding a solution to the cause of this new disease. It was devastating and scaring all of us. I knew my life commitment would be to try to find a solution to AIDS. It has sustained me for 30 years. It continues to be my commitment, and I won't study anything other than AIDS. I will continue to study AIDS until it is gone or I am gone. I am looking forward to studying it today. If you follow your heart and do something that ignites not one, but all of your passion, 100%, you will love medicine every day for the rest of your life. It ignites my passion for discovery, it ignites my passion to connect with my community, it ignites my passion to have an impact ton the world, and it just makes me fully engaged. The lesson may be to follow your heart, and you may not be able to predict what career you will go into, but if you follow your heart you will be fulfilled.

A lens into your life - Have many mentors, advisors, maybe find a life coach, and maybe your patients will be able to give you advice too. Mentors form your education experience, they give you advice. Take or leave that advice, but try to make the most of it. You don't necessarily have to do everything people suggest that you do. Also, patients have this view of physicians that we [physicians] know a lot. The patient knows more about his or her disease, the patient has a theory, the patient him or herself understands what hurts, what doesn't hurt. These other aspects of their own experience of the disease matter a lot to me. Patient and physician. I think, need more of an advisor, mentor-mentee role across medicine. Sometimes it switches, when the patients teach me things. I learn things about their disease that I didn't know before, something that will help me treat them better and allow me to treat others better as well. Patients teach me how to practice better medicine. It is different between the outpatient and inpatient settings, and there are different kinds of medical relationships. I like it when physicians feel comfortable stepping down from the sacred altar of medical knowledge. [Matt: Like firemen?] Let's celebrate firemen. Put out the fire of disease. Firemen are really cool, they are so brave and courageous, driven by a sense of duty. I sometimes interact with fireman actually. They don't ask questions about whether we should respond to this fire or not. If there is a fire, firemen feel compelled to fight it. It is an automatic response. They call me, and I go. That was the experience as a country physician, not: I call you back, check my schedule and your insurance. They call me, and I go. I wanted to be a fireman actually. Getting to be the physician is a very special and fun role to play. Medicine is not for everyone. People who are drawn to healing and drawn to be part of the health care system can find many roles. Some should be physicians, and others should be nurses and respiratory therapists, social workers and administrative assistants, phlebotomists. A career in health care will really allow your life to be an even greater joy from your greatest days today. It's a gift.

Victor Dzau

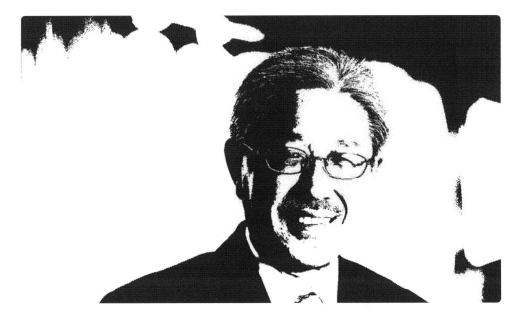

Victor Dzau, M.D. is Chancellor for Health Affairs at Duke University and President and CEO of the Duke University Health System.

our white coat – Several years ago, white coats were a symbol, and were meant for cleanliness and hygiene. Healthcare providers would come from the street and put on their white coat – it would keep them clean. It would also share the symbol of cleanliness of the hospital, and a symbol of knowledge, compassion, purity. A purity of intentions- the fact that it is really important for healthcare providers who

took the Hippocratic oath to put their patients' interests first. I think increasingly the white coat no longer holds the high symbolism that it used to.

While the coat is meant for hygienic purposes more than anything else, sometimes it creates a separation between patient and physician. It sometimes creates an image of "I am the doctor, the most everything, the authority." I am sure you have heard the saying: "the white coat syndrome" that is related to increased patient anxiety when they see their doctors. In fact, to make children feel more comfortable, a lot of pediatricians don't wear white coats.

More and more there is a relationship in medicine (separate from white coats) between physicians and patients that is a more level playing field. Patients have rights, their own intelligence, they want to partner with the physician in terms of their health. To maintain hygiene and minimize infection, it is more important to wash our hands and wear clean clothes. Sometimes I'll walk into a store and see people wearing surgical gowns and white coats, is that really what they are meant for?

attending to the world – We always have to remind ourselves and our trainees, physicians are there to serve. When you serve, you are attending to the patients and their families and to society. Sometimes you forget that. It could be construed in different ways. At the end of the day, the principal reason that physicians and all healthcare providers exist is for those who need their services. To care for the sick, for disease prevention, and to eliminate any kind of health disparities.

a loving smile – I think your themes "the white coat," "attending to the world," and "a loving smile" all speak to the importance of physicians' commitment to patients and service. A healthy relationship between care provider and patients requires a level of trust, a level of chemistry, a level of interaction. A smile is a very important thing. It certainly does not put a separation

between a physician and patient, it is a warm and welcoming gesture. One should almost always have a smile.

Of course a smile is not always appropriate for all situations, e.g. when patients are dying or when a physician is speaking to the family of a patient who has passed. A smile disarms the patient, it makes them feel welcome, and levels the playing field. For years, physicians were trained with the attitude that because they have to make judgments objectively, there must be an "emotional" separation between them and the patients. However, we all recognize these days that patients are our partners. A level playing field is very important. Patients feel vulnerable and stressed when they seek medical care. So, we must wear a warm smile and make them feel comfortable. And it is important for them to have the opportunity to partner with their physician in making many important decisions.

a life apart – We have to really make a serious effort to not have the separation. Objective judgments are always necessary to be a good physician. Yet, we must repeatedly level the playing field. The practice of medicine is an art as well as science. You have to be highly compassionate, and collegial, and on the other hand, you have to have objectivity. That objectivity is the "life apart" issue that you've been talking about. The doctor patient gap should be much, much smaller, yet the ethical objective has to be maintained that requires an emotional apartness for what we need to do.

a lens - One has many images and many experiences in one's life. These inspire you to a great level. I am a physician-scientist. Yet, my role is not only seeing patients and doing research, I am an administrator as well, and in that role I also see how we can make the environment better for our trainees, our providers, and importantly for our patients. One always remembers one's life experiences as a physician.

For me, I remember a forty-year-old with heart failure. He was severely short of breath, and in those days there were no drugs specifically for his condition. It was the late 1970's. While there was a limited quantity of drugs we could use, including digitalis and diuretic, which were helpful but limited in effectiveness. We had a great desire to do more but had few options. We did the very best to reduce the symptoms and make him comfortable, but wanted to do more.

As a physician scientist, I was inspired by the quest to find better treatment and solutions for our patients in need. In doing research, I felt that I would have that opportunity to a make a difference. At that time I was beginning to do research on angiotensin and ACE, which turned out to be an underlying cause for heart failure condition. I was working with a professor at Harvard who was synthesizing new inhibitors to ACE and we administered the ACE inhibitor to this patient under an experimental protocol. It turns out by doing very early research,

we were able to save this man's life; a week later he was able to leave the hospital.

The day I discharged him, under an experimental drug that made him look so much better, I believed he didn't have much means.

I went up to him and said, "Mr. X , would you like some money for a taxi home?" I was going to give him some money. He reached into his pocket and had rolls of 10's and 20's. He said, "Doc, I am okay for cash." It turned out that his condition improved enough for him to have played cards with the other patients and won. Quite amazing how he went from being so sick to winning at cards.

You can think about cancer patients, young pediatric patients, it is a a really rewarding life where you can make a difference. You can advance the way in which you can treat others.

Something very important in my life is translation. It is science that can make a difference to treatments. I grew up in post-war China. I also observed a lot of people in poverty and illness, some of the illnesses affected my own family. I was very influenced by my experience on health disparities. So I am very involved in global health and community health but remain true to my great commitment to doing research and caring for patients. If you combine those passions with science, what you may bring together is a complete look at how one can improve healthcare, in this country and globally.

Wiley Souba

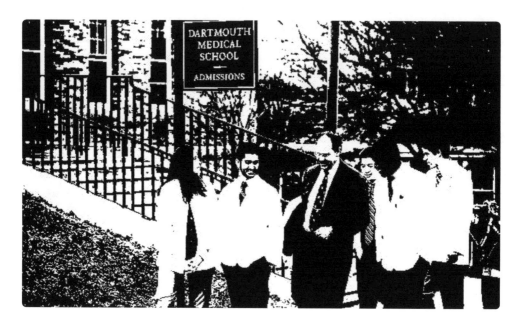

Wiley Souba Jr., M.D. is Dean of Geisel School of Medicine at Dartmouth.

our white coat - The white coat has been the most well-known and visible symbol of the "physician as healer" for centuries. It is also emblematic of the inviolability of doctor-patient relationship. The color white stands for purity, wholeness, and freedom from illness and suffering. This is crucial today when the medical profession is being challenged along the entire range of its cultural values and its traditional roles and responsibilities. The best physicians help their patients rewrite their illness narratives so they can rise above their circumstances and undergo healing.

attending to the world - Our best attending physicians in academic medicine recognize that they serve multiple communities: patients (and their families), students, residents, and colleagues. In serving their patients, their health and well-being must always be the focus of their attention regardless of their social status or ability to pay. Physicians must also be exemplary role models. Behaviors – good and bad –

are emulated and powerfully shape the organizational culture.

The understanding that each of us has of the physician-patient relationship will impact greatly how we approach the care of our patients. If the relationship is viewed solely as a contract for services rendered, the law and the courts prevail; if it is viewed merely as applied biology, it is governed by science; if it is approached exclusively as a commercially driven business transaction, it is regulated by the marketplace. If, however, our relationship with our patients reaches beyond the "delivery" of care to one that is seen as a covenant in which we act in the patient's best interest no matter what, it is based on trust and commitment. It is from this kind of relationship that you will experience the profound joy associated with being a doctor.

a loving smile - The human smile is the most universal of all greetings. It says "Welcome, I acknowledge you and accept you." It attaches profound meaning to the shared bond of all humanity. Even under the toughest of circumstances, the caregiver's smile embodies caring, fosters trust, and symbolizes the physician's commitment to her or his patient.

a life apart - Your effectiveness as a physician is largely a function of your moment to moment way of being. And, there are times when being sad is your natural self-expression. Patients want their physicians to be naturally self-expressed –

they want to experience their doctors as human beings. When you're naturally self-expressed, you always bring your "A" game!

a story - Nearly all of our medical students at the Geisel School of Medicine participate voluntarily in at least one community service project. This is an opportunity for them to take care of the least fortunate among us and establish a relationship with their patients and often their patients' families. They visit their communities and listen to their life story. Invariably, the students report that they receive much more than they give. Whenever you commit to a future bigger than yourself, the rewards are incredible.

William Brody

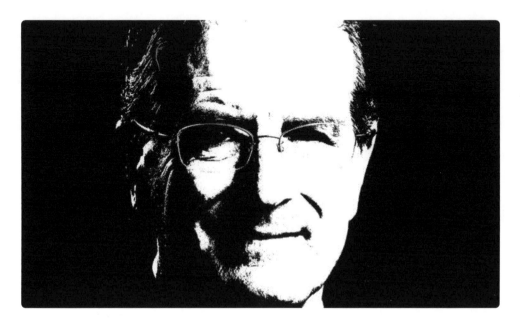

William Brody M.D., Ph.D. is President and Irwin Jacobs Presidential Chair at the Salk Institute.

our white coat - Well, I think that patients play a major role in the healing process. I would recommend that students read Anatomy of Hope by Gerome Grutman who details the patient-doctor relationship within this process extremely well - one of my all-time favorites. He talks about his experiences as a physician and relates some amazing things about the healing process, which he had no concept of when he finished medical school. He realized that the modulation of disease can be affected in a major way by psychology, patient participation in the decision-making process, and patient willingness to undergo treatment. I think that the doctor-patient relationship used to always start with the doctor on a pedestal and the patient in a passive role. The more we learn about making this process effective, the more we learn that it has to be a partnership of equals. You know, not always and not completely in a uniform sense, but I personally believe that patients need to be given a stronger role in their diagnosis and treatment, and doctors need to actively form a better partnership with each of their patients. And the ubiquitous nature of information these days makes it easier for the patient to be informed. In other countries, when you go to the hospital, the patient's family plays a role in the care of the patient, providing meals and some of the nursing care. A lot of these concepts are becoming recognized by mainstream and Western-oriented healthcare. Between the patient and the doctor wearing the white coat, there definitely should be a shared experience. However, this is not easily accepted by all members of the profession, and there is an increasing divide, in part, due to technology that is not in the best interest of our patients.

attending to the world - I think that is the essence of being a physician. You are a servant to other human beings. The question is where does that stop, particularly when you add a financial payment to the equation. It is a lot easier in many other countries where physicians are salaried and where the care is paid by the government. In the United States, finances often get in the way, particularly when physicians graduate with a lot of debt. The level of remuneration becomes a challenge, quite frankly, because Medicaid and Medicare depend on the type of physician. The fact that we do not compensate for the fixed expense gets in the way of these ideals of serving humanity.

uplifting the medically underserved - I'm not sure what it means for something to be a right.

Society has an obligation to provide for its citizens in ways that the society itself deems appropriate. It really depends on the particular society. The real travesty is that, despite the fact that we spend twice as much on healthcare as other nations, we fail to provide some sort of safety net for all of our citizens. We are unique amongst our peers. The United States has an ethical obligation to provide healthcare and, I believe, to a large extent health, to all of its citizens. Is that true of Bangladesh or China? Well, that becomes a complicated equation. Certainly, in the United States, there is no reason that we should not have some form of universal coverage, even if it is not as complete and comprehensive, as some people might like. Even the Affordable Care Act is not intended to provide uniform, universal coverage for everybody. The challenge for our country is that you really need to distribute the three trillion dollars in lives rather than in political reverence. My father was a physician in the era before Medicare and Medicaid. He and his peers volunteered their time at the county hospital, and he had a number of patients from whom he never charged anything. That was a time when medical care was simpler, and we were not talking about chemotherapy with a $100,000 cost per year or complicated ICU treatments. In some ways, when the government steps in to provide coverage, it pushes out other mechanisms by which society has figured out how to provide coverage and make an impact for the medically underserved. It is still imperfect, even in a government-run system. Studies show that most Medicare beneficiaries are happy. Physicians are not all that happy. In total, it is probably a good thing. There are so many people living longer that the healthcare system for senior citizens that existed before just cannot reasonably be considered effective.

a loving smile - I cannot say that I am appropriately qualified to answer this question. Bonding does not necessarily mean hugging or touching in a social way. It is finding an appropriate way to communicate with a patient. The big travesty right now is that we have so pushed the cost equation that physicians are spending even less time with patients than they did before. This is particularly true and unfortunate in the primary care setting. Allowing physicians to spend more time with their patients would actually reduce medical costs. One needs to compensate primary care physicians in a different way and in a higher way in order to allow them to spend more time with patients.

a story - I have a friend, a colleague, named Sanford Greenberg. He goes by the nickname Sandy. Sandy went to Columbia University in the 1950's on scholarship and his roommates were on scholarships there as well. He came from a rather poor family. His sophomore year in college he became blind. One of his roommates read his textbooks to him every night. You can imagine being in college and losing your sight before the age of computers and speech translation devices. Then you can imagine (having been pre-med yourself), it would

take a lot of time to read textbooks to your roommate every night. Would you take the time? Sandy graduated from Columbia University with highest honors and won the Rhodes Scholarship to study at Oxford. Sandy managed to save up $300 in his bank account while he was at Oxford. One day, he received a call from his former roommate, who said, "I am dropping out of college and I want to sing, I want to become a professional musician. I am told we have to cut a record. My parents think this is a terrible idea so they will not help me with the money for it." Sandy took his life savings and gave it to his roommate. His roommate was Art Garfunkel of Simon & Garfunkel. He played at Sandy's wedding thirty years later, and I had the privilege of attending. People who give a lot always say that they get more than they give. A number of people at Johns Hopkins and here at Salk have told me that.

Faculty and Community Leaders

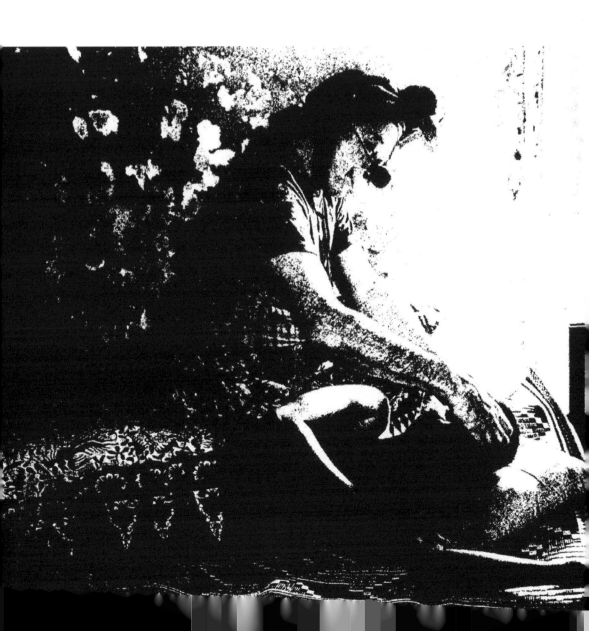

Andru Ziwasimon-Zeller

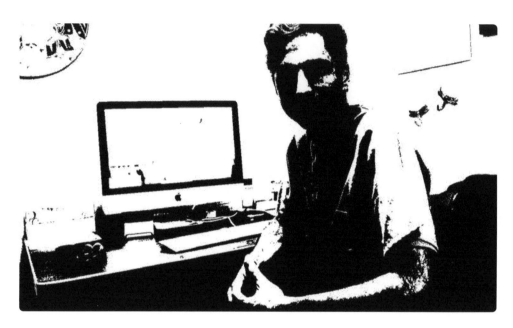

Andru Ziwasimon-Zeller M.D. is Co-Founder of the Casa de Salud Medical Office in Albuquerque, New Mexico, a clinic geared towards serving low-income and uninsured patients. He is also a National Robert Wood Johnson Community Health Leader award winner.

our white coat - Healing is a process of knitting back together a substance that has been rent asunder: body tissue, heart energy, family, society. A doctor can set the context for healing or poison it. Patients can embrace the opportunity with courage and trust, or hold their breath and hide. Healing is the magic of the moment when the wound is no longer alone, confused, ignored. It is when doctor and patient glimpse each other's humanity, with attention and care-each in different roles, for that moment.

attending to the world - If all I did was push my world of birth and place onto others with authority, I would not have a meaningful impact. Instead, a balance of receive and share opens worlds of insight and knowledge. Promoting health then shifts, a better fit, and people hear their own wise words with my voice.

a life apart - When a truth of suffering enters the room and I am the first to name it, before I share this news, I sometimes let myself grieve for pain and loss in the silence of that moment. Moving forward is important; it is not my grief to dwell in.

a story - I was fresh out of residency working alone in a rural ER. A women was brought in by her grown daughter - hallucinating, drunk, long psychiatric story. After the nurse left, we cared for her as if there was no hospital. Haldol and restraints were replaced with an acceptance of her shrieks and moans that shifted over 20 minutes to breath and language. The woman broke her storm and shared her grief of a childhood filled with sexual abuse by her grandfather and her father; this was a new disclosure. I didn't ship her to the psych hospital. She walked out with her family in the morning, ready to seek a Spiritual Healer. A long road ahead but at least she had her foot upon a path, her shrieks of outrage and betrayal no longer confused with schizophrenia. I hope she has found some peace.

Amy Rezak

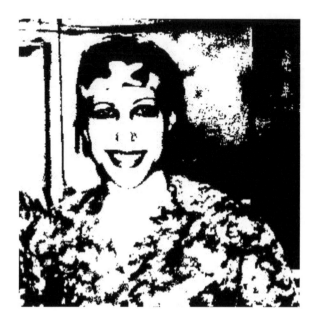

Amy Rezak, M.D. is a Captain of Trauma Surgery for the United States Army and an Assistant Professor of Surgery at the University of North Carolina School of Medicine.

Dr. Rezak was also the star of ABC's hit documentary series *BostonMed* as a Trauma Surgical Fellow at Brigham and Woman's Hospital in Boston. Dr. Rezak is a veteran of the Iraq War.

our white coat - I believe that the white coat represents hope, trust, knowledge, and security. Patients and their families have hope or faith that "the white coat" can help them. However, it is not uncommon for patients, their families, or society to become blinded by the coat and forget that we too are only human. Therefore, I see it as my obligation to help them keep that hope and faith, yet at the same time set realistic expectations.

attending to the world - I had the opportunity to learn medicine in a third world country. I was humbled by my experience there and will never forget how fortunate I am. That said, I do feel obligated, no matter where I am, to help during an emergency.

a loving smile - Because of the nature of my specialty, I often get to know my patients AFTER I have operated on them. One thing I try to remember is that patients know their bodies better than anyone, even doctors. I try to be straightforward and honest yet not too serious. I treat them how I would want someone to treat my family. I really enjoy watching their progress and getting to know them. I have to admit, this is one of the most rewarding parts of my job.

a life apart - I think at this point in my career, with respect to my feelings, I have become completely numb to death and critical illness. Some may view this as being insensitive, but I view this as having the strength to be able to help people despite the severity of the illness. I have witnessed many horrific and tragic events during my career, so I tend to use humor as a coping mechanism.

a story - I was a fourth year medical student on the first day of my general surgery clerkship. The surgical residents chose their cases for the day, advised us to do the same and went off to the operating room. I noticed that one case, a tonsillectomy, was left uncovered by the residents so I chose that. The Attending welcomed me into his room and told me that residents don't usually cover his cases. He proceeded to test my knowledge on anatomy and the current procedure. He then allowed me to perform the procedure (under very close supervision). That was the day I chose surgery as my specialty.

a lens - In the attached photo, I just finished operating for the day at Camp Ramadi, Iraq.

Arnold Gold

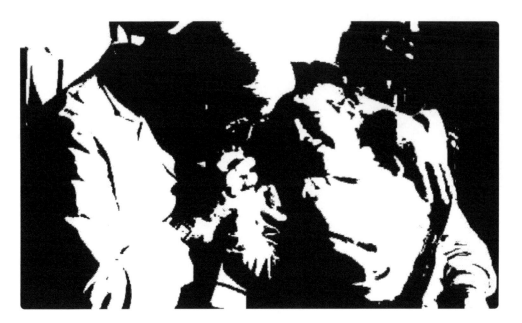

Arnold P. Gold, M.D. is Professor of Clinical Neurology and Pediatric Neurology at Columbia University College of Physicians and Surgeons. The Arnold P. Gold Foundation, a not-for-profit whose mission is to "perpetuate the tradition of the caring doctor," is named in his honor.

our white coat - I helped to create the white coat ceremony. The white coat ceremony developed from the medical school graduation of the Columbia College of Surgeons and Physicians. After everyone receives his or her diploma typically the class stands up and recites the Hippocratic Oath or some oath that defines what kind of doctor he or she will become, in the presence of family and meaningful others as well as in the presence of faculty. At that time they will receive their white coat. I heard students take the Hippocratic Oath and said to myself, this is four years too late, they are already the doctors they are going to be. They should make an oath on the first day and not on the last day, in the presence of their families and the faculty of medicine to tell everyone what kind of doctor they will be, a firm oath to never forget human suffering. And when this happens, as appreciation and recognition a white coat is then given and each student is cloaked in his or hers. Hopefully this white coat is a daily reminder of the oath that they took on entering medical school. The white coat is just a symbol and is not the essence of the white coat ceremony. The essence is the oath.

Wearing the white coat as a physician is just to recognize that this is someone who is to alleviate human suffering and who will establish a relationship with a patient and his or her family. It could be a grey coat or any color, I happen to believe that white is, in at least my mind, a symbol of purity and cleanliness. I don't think it is a barrier, rather a valuable asset that helps to cement a relationship with a patient.

When one enters the field of medicine, as a medical student, and subsequently as a practitioner, service is essential. You are there to serve your patient, you are there to understand his or her suffering. So the essential ingredient is that there is a doctor-patient relationship and that you are serving the patient. Hopefully with the importance of service, most and all will be dedicated to being there for each patient and to society. I do believe that if there is a central focus of service, you will never be negative about practicing medicine. There will be great gratification. Being an agent of service you don't have burnout, you love being a doctor, and there is a great deal of inner satisfaction. This itself enhances emotional stability and happiness, so I do believe that service is an essen-

tial ingredient in being a physician both medically and socially.

attending to the world - I love being a doctor, I have been a doctor for close to 60 years at the Columbia College of Physicians and Surgeons. I enjoy waking up as I go into the subway under the George Washington Bridge. I experience real excitement every day as I am about to have the privilege of hearing my patient's story and hopefully responding to it in a positive manner. I enjoy from the moment I get up till I cross the bridge into Manhattan; at the end of the day as the sun sets, I am exhilarated. With all the problems with the health system and medicine, it is still the greatest profession. I enjoy teaching, practicing, and writing about medicine. All these areas have been very gratifying. And I enjoy medicine as if it were my first day.

[Matt]: "You're so inspiring."

I don't know whether I'm inspiring. If you establish relationships, relationship care, trust that is 100% mutual honesty, you too will receive the gift of practicing medicine, and it will be very satisfying.

a loving smile - When I start with a new patient, it is important to establish a relationship with the child as well as his or her family. I hopefully with effective communication, both body language and spoken communication- the right manner, trust, respect, and honesty must be mutual- will have parents who trust me and be honest with me as I wish them. If we have that, we do bond with one and other. No matter what the scenario, I'm hopefully a change agent and improve the health and welfare of each of my children. I love children, hopefully I relate well to all children as they relate to me. If a child cries I consider myself a failure. No child should cry in my office. Hopefully, if we can establish a relationship, it will be an experience of joy for child and his or her family. Bonding with the child and of equal importance bonding with the family are essential to being an effective clinician.

a story - My favorite story in medicine was when I was an intern at Charity Hospital in New Orleans, an affiliate of Tulane University and Louisiana State. Doing a rotating internship, my first rotation was infectious diseases, and I reported on July 1 to enter my internship. I found that there was a ward full of 35 infected children with polio. Many of them were in iron lungs because they didn't have respirators at that time. The Attending, Margaret Smith, was my first real mentor - I learned always from my teachers, they helped fashion me in the way I am today. She stayed in the hospital for the entire day and night, she didn't go home ever. She remained at the bedside of these children in iron lungs. I just automatically assumed that the interns should do the same thing. So I remained with her 24/7 during the month of internship.

It changed my life. It made me recognize the importance of relationship-centered care. A re-

lationship with patients and relationship with my teachers. I didn't plan on going into Pediatrics. Dr. Smith changed all of that for me. The importance and joy for relating to a child, his or her family, changed my whole life. Each medical student should look for mentors that will help develop their love for medicine. Dr. Smith was one of them. I did my residency with Dr. Ashley Weech (Chair of the Department of Pediatrics at Cincinnati Children's Hospital). Sidney Carter was my mentor at Columbia College of Surgeons and Physicians. These three mentors were the people who made me the kind of doctor that I am today. Look for doctors that you would tend to relate to and hopefully they will have an impact on your practice of medicine. Each played a significant role in developing and enjoying an importance of relationship centered care. I enjoy teaching, teaching residents, both the academic areas and the clinical areas. I developed with these mentors. Each student hopefully will build a relationship that will help fashion what kind of physician he or she will become.

a lens - I also have a foundation, the Arnold P. Gold Foundation. This was the name that the Board of Trustees felt it should be, as they felt my patients would support it, which they did. Twenty-five years in existence, I am certain it has changed the culture of medicine through its many, many programs. It's signature program being the white coat ceremony, the student clinician ceremony. It has also been very important in giving grants to students who can do summer fellowships as well as resident and practicing physicians. The Gold Foundation, I do believe, has impacted our medical education at all levels and helped change the culture of medicine. For the last 25 years, it has been my principal interest aside from my patients.

We also have a humanism honor society, with 103 chapters, which is still developing. It emphasizes the importance of medicine and clinical excellence. You want someone who is at the cutting-edge of medicine and highly proficient. At the same time, without humanism you are not a complete doctor. Humanism is one end and clinical excellence is on the other hand. I couldn't have done this without my wife Sandra, who has been the engine that kept us in the forefront of developing programs related to humanism.

Atilla Uner

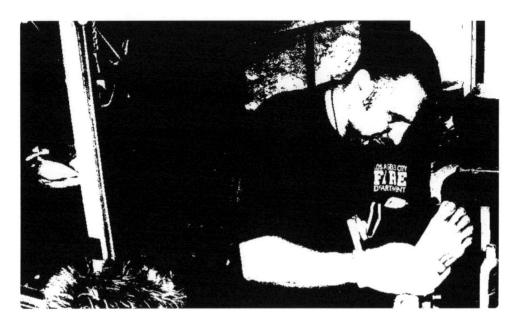

Atilla Under M.D. is Associate Medical Director at the UCLA Center for Prehospital Care; Tactical Medicine Physician for the Hawthorne Police Department; Medical Team Manager, FEMA Urban Search and Rescue California Task Force 2; and Associate Professor of Emergency Medicine at the David Geffen School of Medicine at UCLA.

attending to the world - Being a physician is a very privileged position. We enjoy immediate trust and authority with our patients. Patients will open up to you and divulge things that they would not share with any other human being. We see them when they are in distress and when all their defenses are down. I started as a medic on an ambulance, and I found this access to people very enriching and enlightening. I learn from my patients through learning about their perspectives on life.

Medicine is a service to others at it's very core. Basic medical interventions such as draining an abscess or splinting a fracture involve touching, manipulating, direct physical contact and one-on-one communication. We are helpers and counselors to our patients, no matter what walk of life they have chosen.

uplifting the medically underserved - Healthcare equity is just a small part of what humans should all enjoy: A life as a free person, free from oppression, coercion, violence, and manipulation. For this we need essential political rights such as freedom of speech, freedom of assembly, freedom to move and travel, the pursuit of happiness, and absence of tyranny. Access to education, participation in the political process, and the ability to live a dignified life will follow if the society we live in is free and open. Equal opportunity leads to equity in access. Access to healthcare is but a small facet of the ideal of individual liberty and a dignified existence.

a life apart - It is always okay to feel saddened if the situation you are encountering elicits that feeling in you. But realize that a sad physician doesn't help anyone. Patients and their families entrust us with their most precious good when in distress, their own or their loved one's life and health. They need and deserve a competent, calm, sincere, empathetic partner and advocate who can function with authority and aplomb when they are unable to cope. All physicians react differently to a medical event in their own family or among their friends than when they are doing their medical work. We maintain an inner distance to the event so that we can function when our patients cannot.

a loving smile - Patients want a professional to help them in their time of distress, and they want that person to be friendly, sincere, and understanding. Bonding should mean that we genuinely like our patients, even if their faults and biases are different from our own.

a story - I was a junior EMT and on one of my first ride-along shift with a senior EMT crew on an ambulance in Munich, Germany. We were called to a "person down". When we arrived we found a man on the sidewalk, actively seizing. My mentors attended to the patient and asked me to get the gurney from the ambulance. I was shaking so much I could not function. I was barely able to get the gurney. Meanwhile, my colleagues, unperturbed, calmed down bystanders, obtained IV access, determined blood sugar, secured the patient whose seizure had now stopped onto the gurney, loaded the patient into the ambulance, and made radio contact. How could they be so calm when everything else was falling apart? What enabled them to take charge, bring order to chaos, and fix what was broken? Surely, their education and skills must have allowed them to assess, prioritize, and act effectively. I wanted to learn how to master situations that were so frightening to me and the other onlookers. Medicine has allowed me to do just that. It is a wonderful profession.

a lens into your life - I really don't have an average day because I have so many assignments. I serve as an emergency department physician at a community hospital and at an academic medical center. I teach emergency medicine to students, physicians in training, nurses and paramedics. Not having an average day is what keeps me alive more than anything. Medical supervision of care delivered in ambulances and helicopters is my public health involvement; it is pro bono work, I don't get paid for the majority of it. I enjoy interacting with people who are actually doing the hands-on work, and helping the those who ask me, "Hey Doc, I had this perplexing case last week in the field, maybe you have an explanation for what happened there?" Public health and medical care don't just happen, they are provided by people who deserve a physician to support them. Mentoring is the role that I enjoy most.

Bernie Siegel

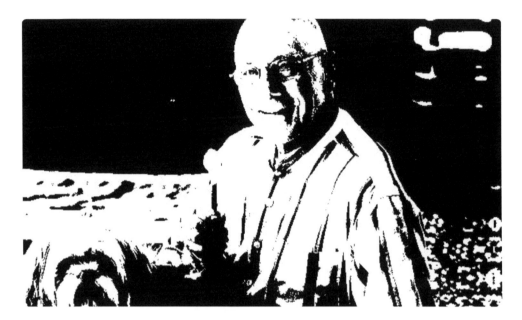

Bernie Siegel M.D. is Author of the New York Times #1 Bestselling Book, *Love, Medicine, and Miracles,* and Professor Emeritus in the Department of Surgery at Yale University School of Medicine.

our white coat - "Why did you become a doctor?" I always ask students,and, "Why are you thinking of a certain specialty, and who is focused on health?" I ask students to draw a picture of themselves working as a doctor, as I think a visual response to these questions is often most sincere. Most students draw themselves sitting at a desk with a diploma on the wall. Many draw lots of instruments. Maybe if they all go into research, they will be ok. One of my students who impressed me was one who drew himself kneeling in front of a woman in a wheel chair and handing her a tissue. He is touching her as a human being. To the question "Why did you become a surgeon?" I answer, "I became a surgeon as a reaction formation to my destructive tendencies, I love cutting people open, and I didn't want to end up in jail." I do this so people will think about their healthy and unhealthy reasons for becoming a doctor. We need to change the culture. People come in the bodies we are caring for.

I once wrote to the Dean of Weill Cornell Medical College, my alma matter. It took over 50 years for anyone to respond to me. Each time a new dean took over during the past five decades, I sent in another copy of my letter. My letter discussed how they never taught me to take care of people, and what I thought needed to be amended in the Weill Cornell Medical College curriculum. I couldn't believe it took 50 years to receive a response, not even a form letter for five decades. This shows how sick our system is. Students receive medical information, not a medical education at most institutions. Right now we treat disease, we don't treat people.

Now, more specifically with regard to the physical white coat, it is a relationship that is what it is about. To me when I think of my white coat, I think of a blank canvas. If you are creating a painting and do not like the way that it looks, you correct it, you touch it up. You don't simply say it is no good and throw it out. We need to correct the patient-doctor relationship. We need to step back and look at this from a wider angle. Doctors are inherently always looking at disease, and patients are inherently always looking for that relationship. I often ask people what are you experiencing and not what is your diagnosis. By helping them with their experiences, I also help them to heal their lives. The white coat at the end of the day is a symbol of purity and spirituality. It is all the colors, like the rainbow Never forget it is the po-

tential of the blank canvas, and you have the opportunity to create so many meaningful, truly beautiful relationships with every patient you see.

I feel it is meaningful to also share a personal story in response to this theme. My father in-law was a quadriplegic whose forehead itched. When he recently went to the hospital, they gave him medication which put him to sleep. When they could have scratched his forehead instead of making his life meaningless. As a physician, I ask that you never forget to put that line in; it is so simple, "What is going on in your life?" and "What are you experiencing? before you grab the prescription pad or syringe. The words they answer with will relate to their life experience too.

I made a living at my life in medicine, yeah. But I didn't keep track of who paid me. I didn't worry whether people paid, didn't pay. If I had enough to go home and feed the family, fine. For other doctors it was different. One time a colleague bumped into my car in the Yale University School of Medicine parking lot. I told him, "I will get it fixed and tell you how much it costs, would that be okay with you?" He started screaming at me, not about the car, about how he operated on my child and I never paid him. I told him I would look into it and called the insurance company. They said they mailed me a check but it was never cashed. So they sent another and I gave it to him. I found it sad, he was keeping track of the fact his own friend didn't pay him. I would have paid the bill if he just asked about it. Instead, he kept it inside, resenting me and I didn't know what was going on. When patients came in, I took care of them.

Our white coat is really about deceiving people into good health. Matthew, you'll learn basically that hypnotic techniques can help you talk to people in a way that calms them. If we were trained to talk to people, we could accomplish so much more. What the doctor says doesn't have to be true as long as it is ethical. I had a patient who got mad instead of getting depressed when the doctor told him he wouldn't see the sun come up the next day. I had another patient look at his chart, see the words "doing well", and respond to his doctor's words. I may add, write the word down several times , without spaces and they become swords. What do you see, Matthew? Here, try it. The words become a swords. You can literally kill people with your words or a scalpel similarly.

Similarly, I had a patient who was nervous about going into surgery. She nervously said, "Thank God for all these wonderful people." I replied, "I have worked with them for years they're not wonderful people," She started laughing,we became family and her fear was gone. I worked with them for years and they knew my technique and sense of humor. It's always important to stand up for what you believe in when stuff like this happens. Everyone here at Yale expects those crazy comments from me on the surgery floor. I do all kinds of crazy stuff, like talk to patients when they are under anesthesia, and I credit myself with being the first to play music in the operating room. Other surgeons agree; ask them. Finally, they realized it benefited patients to have surgeons and staff be relaxed. That is what I say to all the Yale University medical students; if you know something works, just do it, and tell stories about it. If you tell a case history, or an anecdote, people don't feel threatened, they listen, and they learn from it. Ok, so let me tell you how this worked. I brought my tape recorder into the operating room. They said it was an explosion hazard. I still brought it in. Within a week, patients all felt better listening to music. In a month or two, all the surgeons at Yale University School of Medicine had their little boom boxes playing tapes. Look at this, I mean WOW, everyone was feeling better and everyone was doing it. Operations were shorter, patients needed less anesthesia and had less pain. Once it got accepted, then of course you had people doing studies and what not. Before it was accepted, no one would go fund a study on something like this. I mean, Matthew, I'm not encouraging you to go blow up hospitals, but if you find something simple and meaningful, it could work you know.

Oh and also, students would shadow me for a month from my house to the operating room. They would eat some breakfast with me, we would scrub together, and then we would go to the operating room. If I missed something, or I wasn't listening, they knew they were supposed to tell me. It gave them practical experience that they could see what the life of a leading surgeon was like. I was known as the Carl Jungian surgeon, because all the stuff I brought to my practice from him and his work. We become so specialized, house vs. your body. If you have a problem in your house you call the specialist, the plumber, the locksmith whatever you feel like. But you're a unit. Too often it is, "I'm taking care of your kidneys, your heart, your whatever." That doesn't take care of the person. We need to treat the person as a whole entity and not just the pieces.

attending to the world - That's what changed my life. I like people as I said. I told you that, right Matthew? I became a doctor because I care about people! It was even more painful as a surgeon, there were people who had complications of my surgery. Many times I said to people that I would quit, because I felt so bad about what I did, because of a complication. Matthew, when you are a doctor put your ego against the wall. No looking at that computer screen when a patient is in the room. Face your patient, don't have anything between you and your patient. You're a nice kid; I'd feel better in your office than most of the faculty I know. When you not only help them, but believe in them, they live longer lives and don't die when they were supposed to. That is what has kept me going because I saw what began to happen. Everyone would have a story about what changed their life, what they did, what and how it enhanced their ability to survive. I have literally, I'm not kidding, "I wouldn't lie to you right Matthew?" had people go home to die, and then the cancer disappeared. Some left their troubles to God some laughed more. Like

one went to the mountains, and it was so beautiful, he forgot to die. Life is a labor pain, as a doctor, you help people give birth to themselves. The opposite of love is rejection and abuse, what you want people to know is that you love them even though their parents didn't. I was recently paged to see a suicidal teenager who needed surgery. You're my "CD" she would later say. My "Chosen Dad." Be a Chosen Mother or Chosen Dad. Give them return appointments. Let them know that you care.

What was the other point. I also would like to share Harvard students were asked while at Harvard if their parents loved them or not. 98% of those who said no had experienced an illness by middle age. People who smoke, they're not stupid, 900 years ago, Maimonides wrote that if people took as good care of themselves as they do their animals, they would suffer fewer illnesses. You say to an audience, what do you do when your cat develops lung cancer? A few people say stop smoking but more say I'd smoke outdoors so I don't kill my cats. They didn't publish my letter on the fact that it is okay to kill yourself but not your cats. If you get people to love themselves, then they pay attention to the information. If not then they become addicted to everything. Alcohol, food, drugs, sex, everything.

uplifting the medically underserved - Everybody deserves the right to have access to a physician, and not have it based on the ability of their finances and funds. To know that they can go and will be taken care of. You know we are all God's children, and made of divine stuff, and we all deserve that care. You know it is the right thing because then people begin to care about themselves and for themselves and we all then would save money. If every kid grew up with love from his parents as a start, we would save a fortune. A colleague in Australia once said that if everyone in Australia had a dog, they would save hundreds of millions of dollars because of the lower mortality after a heart attack in homes with a dog. All those things are significantly important.

I defined my career by being available to people, and not worried about it from the perspective of compensation. A child falls into the fireplace and is badly burned. We had to use different sharp instruments and needles, and she screamed at me, "I hate you," every day when I took care of her burns. A few years later when she was coming to the office when it was 90 degrees, I said you have a turtleneck on, it is over 90 degrees. She said, "I'm ugly, I'm ugly." Another visit she said I need to get a job this summer. I knew I could get her a job at a nursing home where they had uniforms which exposed her scars. She took the job. And the next time she came into the office, she said nobody noticed her scars. I said, "Madeline when you are giving love you are beautiful." Few years ago, I got a phone call from her, "my father died a few years ago I'm getting married, will you be my father." When we got up to dance at her wedding, she played, "you never let me down, you turned my life around." That is the greatest gift any doctor can ever have.

You can't match that with funds if you know what I mean. When you get involved with people in this way, and care for them, they become your family. You know, I get thanks for things I did 20 or 30 years ago.

a loving smile -I walked into a room in the hospital worried about my patient, as I walked in she asked, "What's wrong?" She said, "The expression on your face is tight and wrinkled."I said I am thinking about how to help you." She said, "Think in the hallway, and smile when you come in here." I could have said "You're the problem, you just calm down." She knew that I cared and listened. You can't be afraid to bring in humor, when you are laughing the transformation happens to you becoming a friend as well. I am a kid in the hospital I tell anesthesiologists to say things in this mindset when putting a patient to sleep. "What will it feel like to go out, patients often ask?" I say you should say, "How did you feel the last time you went out on a date? It will feel like that!"

a story - Wow, you know I have so many stories. The thing that fascinates me is potential - what creation has built into all living things. You can be part of achieving that potential. I believe in self-induced healing because that is the only way healing truly happens. Medical students, think of a rainbow-colored butterfly as part of your treatment plan. Order and transformation. Really, you should. Don't think about prognosis, remissions, or cures alone. When self-induced healing occurs, you learn something. Learn from your patients when they do well, ask them "what did you do?" "How come you didn't die?" Why don't you have any pain?" They will teach you what you can then teach your other patients. We are not taught survival behavior in the classroom or anatomy lab. Why not learn something and keep learning from your patients. Then you will be participating in some amazing things that can happen in a life. I remember nurses saying to me, your patients are refusing pain medications after surgery, even after major surgery. Nurses would say, "They're not hurting." "It's the patient and their attitude," I would tell the nurses, "they see their participatory role being emphasized, their potential to heal themselves."

I have one other great one. You'll love this one, I promise. The mind is all powerful and everything. I had a cohort of patients where the radiation therapy machine did not have any radioactive material in it due to a repair error. Yet, they were getting better. They believed they were being treated, and they responded to their beliefs. Their tumors shrunk. Let me just sum it up by saying, when patients believe they are being a part of the healing process they are, it is really exciting to me.

a lens into your life - I had a near death experience as a four year old choking on a toy. Living things have been important in my life for a long time. Like Schweitzer I have a reverence for life. I made my house into a zoo. The acre and a half yard full of creatures. With the five kids, I had a crew to take care of them. The police

never reported us. It was done out of love, not a psychotic thing. They were family. A big part of why I became a doctor, was simply caring for living things. Albert Schweitzer called it "reverence for life." I have been picking up worms. When I went out on the street to take a walk today, I just picked them up and put them back on the earth. I think I'm kind of neurotic, but I can't help it, every time I take a dog for the walk, I pick up a million worms and save their lives. Thank you Albert, I'm not crazy.

The last points: the best doctors are criticized by patients, nurses and family. They learn from their mistakes and don't make excuses.

And from Helen Keller: Deafness is darker by far than blindness so listen to your family and patients and they will thank you when they hear what they are saying and know what is right for them without you making any comment.

Any student who needs to get in touch with me, can get in touch with me through my website, www.berniesiegelmd.com.

Christine Montross

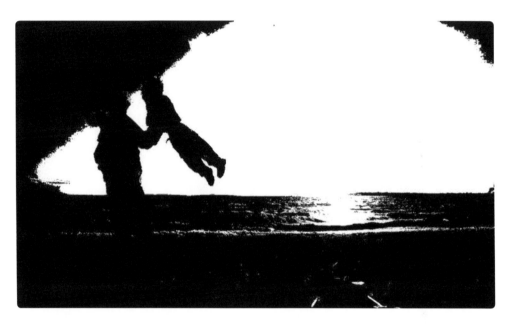

Christine Montrossl M.D. is Assistant Professor of Psychiatry and Human Behavior, Brown University School of Medicine and Bestselling Author, *Body of Work.*

our white coat - It is important for both the physician and the patient to understand and acknowledge the power that the white coat has. As physicians, we lose awareness of that power rather quickly because the coat is a symbol that surrounds us. It's worn by our colleagues—people we perceive to be our equals— and we gradually, imperceptibly lose the view we first had when we put it on. When we first put on the white coat, it feels like it contains a great sense of purpose and responsibility; it continues to have that meaning for our patients, even as its symbolic potency dims for us. We must not to lose sight of that.

Acknowledgment of any element which conveys a difference in power is particularly critical as we are moving toward an understanding that individual health is a team effort. The advice and instruction that we give as physicians is only followed to the degree that the patient not only truly understands it, but also buys into it and agrees with us. Patients are increasingly coming to us with ideas about their own care, and it then becomes our job to determine where those thoughts come from, and whether they have a valid place in the patient's healthcare. It is not our job to dismiss internet research, personal experience, or the experiences of our patients' friends and family members, but to view the information that our patients bring as a means of communicating with us about their concerns, their priorities, and their hopes for their health and their lives.

attending to the world - I think of medicine entirely as a service. People come to us for care, and we aim to provide that care to them as best we can. I love the base word of tend in "attending" because I feel that there is something deep and evocative in that word. Within "attending to our patients," or being "an attending physician," there is the inherent implication that we tend to someone: tend to their needs, tend to their fears. Within the word there is also the thematic link to attention. Increasingly, as medicine moves toward models with greater time constraints on patient-physician interactions, giving attention to our patients in a true, full sense of the word is one of the most meaningful ways in which we can practice.

uplifting the medically underserved - I believe that access to a physician is a basic human right. I have recently been in a position to be able to speak and write about the grave inadequacy of outpatient mental healthcare for the uninsured and the underserved. This has been an opportunity for me to increase awareness for the general public as to the needs that exist, and also to the consequences that occur for all of us when we do not provide adequate care to people. We have a unique and privileged view as physicians. We cannot expect everyone without that view to understand the struggles that our patients endure. As a result, we have a responsibility to share what we see so that others can understand the needs of their fellow citizens. If American voters or lawmakers say that they do not believe that all people have a right to access care, I think we are compelled to speak out, and show those people what that choice looks like; what it means.

a loving smile - Patients come to us in extraordinarily vulnerable positions. They are hurt, or they feel ill, and they need treatment. They are scared by changes in their bodies and need reassurance, or diagnoses, or action. They may be dying. They may have been victimized. In any event, when they come to us they seek care. Warmth and connection put patients and their families at ease. Feeling safe and understood allows our patients to trust more fully that we hear their concerns, that we are calm and rational in the face of their distress, and that we are genuinely embarking with them on a plan for their care.

a story - In my own first year of medical school, I feared that becoming a doctor would necessarily mean giving up certain other aspects of myself that I held dear. I was a writer before I came to medical school, and my biggest fear about medicine was not that I would fail, or that I would not like it. Instead I feared that as a physician I would no longer be able to write. I feared that the demands of the practice of medicine would force me to give up the practice of writing. Yet when I walked into the anatomy lab on that first day, I knew right away that I had to write about my experience there. The experience of human dissection, and the writing that emerged from it, eventually turned into my first book, *Body of Work*. I use that story as an example for first year medical students who are struggling to find balance. One of the real dangers that medical students face is that they can lose sight of the aspects of themselves that they treasure. So I always say to medical students: if you want to be the kind of physician who plays the guitar, or runs races, or visits friends and family, you actually need to begin by being the medical student who does these things. Medicine will take as much time and space as you give it. And it does not get less demanding, though certainly in ways, you have more control over its demands as you progress in the field. You should always keep in mind the kind of doctor you want to be: for me it was a doctor with a full family life, who was also a writer. I encourage students to use medical school as a critical time to begin to practice how to achieve that happy, sustaining balance.

Daniel Lowenstein

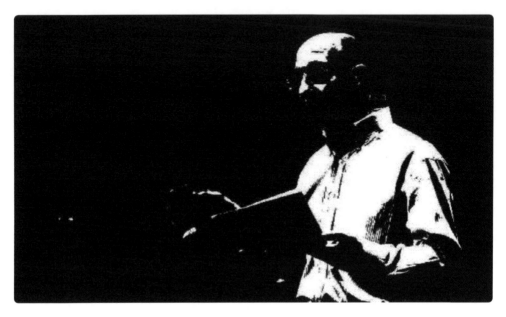

Daniel Lowenstein M.D. is Professor and Vice Chair in the Department of Neurology at UCSF School of Medicine and Director of the UCSF Epilepsy Center.

our white coat -

Bathtime

I.
If you were to ask
about some of my favorite things,
the answer would come simply
without a moment's thought.
"Why, washing my son Stefan's hair,
at bathtime, of course."
It's become
one of those precious rituals
that, thankfully,
both of us have not yet outgrown.

This ritual begins
with a distant call that needs to
prevail over the sound
of crashing, ocean-tub waves,
breach the bathroom door,

reach its way downstairs, and
unearth me from the inertia that comes
from listening to so many distant hollers
from a small parade of children
passing before my eyes.
Children that, despite all the hollering,
still,
could linger as long as they wished.

"Daddy! I'm ready to wash my hair!"

This is the call of the Sirens if there ever was
one.

I always find Stefan sloshing about
in the midst of a never-ending
experiment in fluid mechanics,
self-absorbed,
presumably self-scrubbed,
But the moment he see's me,
the Niagara of questions descend.

"So Dad, what kind of pulleys
should we use in our tram?"
And
"What do you think is a better job -
being someone who designs roller coasters?
Or someone who runs them?"

The questions only stop
when, after placing my left hand
as a cradle
behind his neck,
He leans back and floats

While I hold him with his face
just above the surface of the water.

The questions stop,
because we have both learned well
there's not much point
in holding a conversation
when one's ears
are submerged underwater.

And so, for a time,
he floats, suspended,
while I comb water
through his hair
with my fingers.
All becomes quiet,
all becomes silent.
The surface of the water is an interface that clois-
ters us both from the din
of the world outside.
And Stefan,
serene and silent, floating Stefan,
Looks up with a wide-eyed gaze
at a gloss white ceiling that has become
a movie screen for his dreams.

Here is a place free from the bother
of being told to wear shoes outside,
or finishing homework,
or worrying about tomorrow's
"Mad Minute" arithmetic quiz.
Suspended at the water's surface,
we are both free from
haunting images of the Titanic,
Grandpa's who have gone away,

A friend's mother with cancer,
Planes falling to the ground,
Churches burning in Mississippi,
Explosions in Ireland.

Here is a place where it is quite sufficient
to worry only about
whether the lawn-mower engine-powered airplane
Stefan's decided we will build
should have one seat or two...

II.
My first patient in clinic
is a 23-year old man from Bosnia.
Two years ago,
caught in the crossfire,
a sniper's bullet
grazed his carotid artery just so,
took away the life
in the left side of his body,
and snared his spirit whole.
With crutches, broad shoulders, and powerful
eyes,
wearing his Adidas track suit and running
shoes, he is intent on making it into my room
without help.
My white coat,
safely out of range
beckons him,
directs him to the chair,
examines extraocular movements
and muscle tone

and tendon reflexes.
Moves and arranges
and determines and explains things.
Projects the knowledge and experience of a
very noble profession.

But here
from beneath the surface
of my white coat,
I only see a reflection of myself,
and am overwhelmed
by the reality of his suffering.
I want to imagine him whole again.
Running at full speed
down the soccer field,
I pass him the ball.
His shot is like a bullet,
the crowd roars,
we spin together,
cry out a joyful cry
in celebration of a spectacular goal.

III.
My last patient of the day
is an 80-year old retired physician
from the Republic of Georgia.
Hypertensive, with cardiac disease,
depressed and unsmiling
He came to me a year ago
with unbearable headaches.
He and his grandson,
a loving interpretor,
had greeted my white coat
with great anticipation.

Wanted explanations
about the pathophysiology of his disease,
prognosis,
treatment options.
Thankfully,
the new medication we tried
worked beautifully.
The white coat lived up to its name.

Now, as though a ritual,
he insists on visits
every two months.
As much for our friendship
as for the prescription refills
or blood pressure checks.
Through his grandson he reports
he is still taking long walks that
I have encouraged him to take every day
and he is trying, as best he can, to lose weight.
Reaching through the fabric of my white coat,
He wants to know how my children are doing,
laughs at my jokes,
and reminds me of our plans
to get together and drink some vodka
in celebration of his renewed health.
When he leaves,
his eyes always well up in tears,
he hugs me like a bear,
kisses me on the cheek
as is the custom in Georgia.

IV.
In the finale of the bathtime ritual,
Stefan's face above the water's surface
is surrounded by a halo of shampoo,

as though a living version of one of those Italian
masks you can find in Venice.
Soaking the shampoo out of his hair,
takes time,
must be done gently,
with careful attention to the waterline.
What's the rush anyway?
Stefan,
quiet, silent, floating Stefan,
still seems quite content to soar among his
thoughts.
And I am quite content to watch him.

Finally, when I lift his head up,
the rushing in of the outside world
brings with it the images and sounds
of nuclear tests,
paralyzed gaits,
spectacular goals,
kisses on the cheek, and,
of course,
the unending questions.
"So Dad, what would you rather do?
Climb a mountain or sail a sailboat?"
"Let me think about that for a moment, Stef.
Now, come on now, it's time to get ready for
bed."

a lens into your life -

"UCSF Last Lecture," this has become my most
important piece of work to date:
http://youtu.be/ymAInYRuBOA

David Wofsy

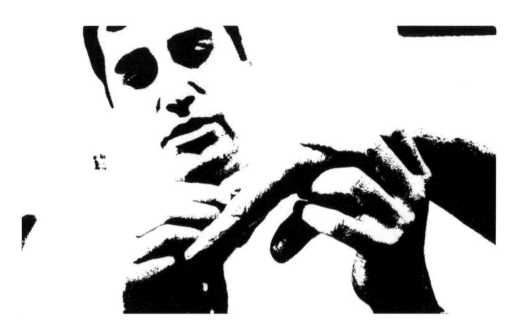

David Wofsy M.D. is Professor of Medicine and Associate Dean for Admissions at the UCSF School of Medicine. He is Past President of the American College of Rheumatology and an attending physician at San Francisco VA Medical Center.

our white coat - I never much cared about what people wear, whether they're people in authority or whether they're patients. We are all equal. Some patients are more comfortable with a doctor who dresses formally and wears a white coat. Some patients are more comfort-able with someone who's more informal. The same goes for physicians. I don't view the garb, either the personal garb or the professional garb, as important determinants of my interaction with people. If I sense that it's important to the patient that I look a certain way, then I'll defer to that. Generally speaking I would prefer not to put a barrier between the patient and myself, but rather to develop a relationship as equals trying to accomplish the same goal.

I think it's very difficult to generalize about medical professionals or about patients. They're all different. Some patients very much want to participate in their care, are capable of doing that, and are equal partners in developing a plan. After all, it's their life, and they should make the best-informed decisions they can. But there is no question that there are other people who feel more comfortable deferring to an expert who has expressed a judgment based on expert education and experience. They feel more comfortable trusting that training and not feeling that they're being pushed to make a decision that they don't feel competent to make. I think one of the challenges of being a good physician is to develop the kind of relationships with people where you can appreciate these differences. We're all human beings. I think what you need to do as a health professional is to be sensitive to different needs. People want to participate in their healthcare in different ways.

attending to the world - Absolutely being a physician inherently means serving another. I think one of the things that physicians have to accept from the beginning is that in situations where their patients have a compelling need, the patient's need has to come over the physican's need. This is something we all accept when we agree to take this responsibility for people's health, to be called in the middle of the night or to be called when you're at a family event. You have to make the judgment that the patient comes first. The responsibility to other people is an inherent part of the profession.

Physicians of today live in a bit of a protected era and environment. Through virtually all of history, doctors exposed themselves to the risk of death when taking care of patients. There was plague, tuberculosis, untreatable communicable diseases of all kinds. People who were physicians knew that they were risking their lives, and often gave their lives, in the service to patients.

It's only very recently in the annals of history that physicians could even begin to have the thought that somehow they shouldn't be vulnerable, that they shouldn't be put at risk for their patients. This may be true during the last 50 years but not before then, and not during the AIDS epidemic, and not in certain parts of the world where it's still true that doctors have to risk their lives when taking care of their patients. It's inherent to the profession to make personal sacrifices for the people we care for, including when there is personal risk.

Are personal relationships the most meaningful part of one's practice?

The broad answer is: people make contributions in different ways in medicine; they derive their satisfaction and sense of value from these different things. Doctors change health care systems; they do research; they do a lot of things that impact patients they'll never meet. I've known colleagues for whom it's all about helping the person in front of them. I would actually extrapolate that beyond medicine. There are many people for whom that's the defining quality: that relationship and ability to make a difference in the life of the person in front of them.

But there are other physicians who have made enormous contributions to the world by doing things that didn't involve relationships with the people they were helping. We have people who develop cures for certain forms of childhood leukemia who will never have relationships with the children whose lives were saved by what they did. But those people will appropriately feel a great sense of satisfaction that's quite independent of direct relationships with patients.

Do I find the greatest satisfaction in the ability to develop a warm and helpful relationship with another human being? Yes, I do. But that's not the only kind of useful life.

uplifting the medically underserved - Access to health care is a human right, but we have seen that the devil is in the details. All of us in the medical field and in leadership positions in society beyond the medical field, have a responsibility to ensure access. It is very well known that we don't do a good job of that in this country. It is our responsibility to improve in that area. It has to be part of the job of everyone who is involved in medicine. Politically speaking, everyone has a stake in the fight for health equity.

Is pursuing health equity the most important goal of a physician who is currently practicing?
Different people find different niches. The world needs the very best neurosurgeon. The world needs someone whose real accomplishment is

exquisite technical skill. Absolutely that person should care about making that skill available independent of means to patients. But should it be their primary interest? Is it the most important thing? For some people the most important thing is something else they contribute. Health equity should be a part of their lives and values. They should strive to contribute to health equity as they can. However, it's perfectly reasonable for it not to be the most important goal for everybody.

a loving smile - It is important to bond with patients. I do think that a warm smile is a particularly important thing in interaction with patients. A sympathetic smile is important. It's crucially important to genuinely care for patients and to communicate that. How you communicate depends on the setting, the severity of illness, and the personality of yourself and of the patient. . There are some people in medicine who serve a vey useful role dong a technical task really well, sometimes involving patients who are unconscious with whom they will never have a bond. We need physicians in these roles, too. But if you're talking about a general picture of a doctor sitting with a conscious patient with a problem, a human bond is crucial.

a life apart - I think the best teaching is done when you're honest, and that means being honest about what you don't know, about what you believe, and about how you feel. I think it's important for students to see that. It is always the case in your personal and professional life that you have to use judgment about the context in which you show emotion and how it will be interpreted, especially if you're in a situation where you're teaching or caring for someone. As a general rule, however, I think it's important to show emotion, to be honest about emotion, to be a human being.

a story - The stories of community health and community responsibility are what I find inspiring. I was a fellow in rheumatology when the first AIDS cases arrived, and what was happening then is that healthy young men were coming in and saying, "I felt fine two weeks ago. Now I have a cough." They had pneumocystis pneumonia, and they were dead two weeks later. All that was clear for quite a while – over a period of three years before HIV was discovered – was that this was communicable, it was invariably fatal, and it could be transmitted to healthcare workers. The people in this institution – and it wasn't everybody, in fact it was a minority of people – who responded properly to that unexpected public health crisis in the community were heroic. In the classic sense of medicine, here was a very frightening epidemic that was happening mostly to people in disenfranchised communities: gay men, IV drug users, prostitutes, racial minorities, poor people. These were the populations that the health care system didn't serve very well even before AIDS came along. So it was not prepared to suddenly serve them well when there was a crisis. By and large, the political community and the health care community responded poorly to the AIDS epidemic, but the doctors who responded properly were inspiring. The fact that this was done well at my institution – a public institution with a public responsibility – was inspiring and was a reflection of what public health and public education were supposed to be about. When I try to tell an inspiring story to applicants to medical school, I often choose the AIDS epidemic because – although not all doctors responded to it properly – the doctors who did really were living out the best tradition of medicine in a very inspiring way.

Then there are the stories of individual patients who have personally inspired me but are harder to communicate to others until you have actually experienced medicine. One of the things that has had a very big impact on me personally has been the opportunity to know and care for people from all walks of life who live and function in realms that don't overlap much with mine – areas of society that I might never encounter if I were not a physician. Personal courage and strength of character exists no matter where you look in society. That's should not be surprising, but it is nonetheless inspiring to see people who are living under the harshest and most challenging circumstances, with comparatively few resources, who rise in a courageous way to the medical problems their family members or they themselves have. That is really inspiring.

[Matt: Were you one of the first responders when the AIDS crisis began?]

The answer is no, but my wife was. She was an Infectious Disease specialist at San Francisco General Hospital, and she literally saw the first two cases of AIDS in San Francisco. So while I wasn't the first responder, I did live with the first responder from the first case to 15 years later when she died of breast cancer. So I felt very close to the AIDS epidemic and the first responders and knew them all very well because of my relationship to her. All of us who were seeing patients in San Francisco at that time were taking care of patients with AIDS, so I certainly had my own firsthand experience and had to deal with my own firsthand fears about the unknown. But it would be a real misinterpretation to count myself among the first responders. The front line got a much, much more challenging experience than I ever had.

[Matt: As we as a country try to fix the healthcare system and provide care for people both who have been disadvantaged by society and simultaneously provide a better system for responding to crises, what are some key ways that you think we could do better as a country?]

Oh, it's hard to even know how to address all of the aspects of society that contribute to poor health and health inequality. While the first temptation is to talk about the healthcare system and the health insurance system, the reality is that it goes much deeper than that. So if you really care about the health of society, you would deal with poverty. You would deal with unequal educational opportunities. You would

deal with the societal issues that have contributed to an increasing gap between the haves and the have-nots, because healthcare problems often reflect that very fundamental inequality that goes way beyond the healthcare system but also dramatically influences access to healthcare. That's really the first issue – that this society has such social and economic inequality that the problems of the healthcare system are virtually inevitable.

That said, the healthcare system itself could do a much better job even in the context of the social challenges. That would begin, in my opinion, with an entirely different approach to health insurance; giving real meaning to the notion that healthcare is a right for everyone; removing the administrative, bureaucratic and economic impediments to people from getting appropriate healthcare. It would take very fundamental change in society to create the kind of healthcare system that most of us in medicine would like to see.

[Matt: As the UCSF Associate Dean for Admissions, you have the opportunity to read hundreds of inspiring personal statements from young people interested in medicine, what inspires you most about the next generation?]

I don't think this generation is fundamentally different than the one I grew up in and probably no different than the one that my parents grew up in. The idealism of youth is a very positive force in the world. And to the extent that people can hold onto it – despite the blows that real life deals to people, the real life challenges that people have to make a priority – the better we are.

[Matt: This question and the different answers we have gotten have scared me a little. It's worrisome to think that perhaps the system isn't changeable.]

The system is changeable. The world changes – it doesn't change at the pace that we want it to change, but the world changes. If you think about the problems that exist today – many of them are traceable to older problems, but it's not hard to see that things have changed. If you're gay in this country, things are very different for you than they were 40 years ago. If you're African American in the South, things are different. There's a long way to go in both of those areas, but it's not difficult for me to look back on my life and see that there have been fundamental changes. Certainly if you look back longer – 100 years, 200 years, 300 years – the world changes. Even at my age, I'm idealistic enough that – although not every single change is a change for the better – the general flow, as long as we don't blow ourselves up, is for the world to become a better place.

[Matt: What do you think allows you to balance such strong humility at the same time with confidence and agency towards making an impact and towards advancing the field and healthcare as a whole?]

That's a very kind and flattering way of asking the question, so it's hard to answer it with-

out sounding arrogant. I think that there are two pieces of that for me. We are all surrounded by people who are capable of things we are not capable of doing. Academic life, if you're honest with yourself, reinforces that perception. I practice medicine part-time because I have a research role and an administrative role. I'm conscious of the fact that people who see patients every day and devote their life to it are doing more good in that realm than I am and are probably better at it; after all, they practice it all the time. Similarly, the people who devote their whole life to science do better science than I do. So I think that most of us recognize we have a narrow range of talent compared to the talents we value. This is true even within our chosen profession and very limited area of expertise, but it is even more evident if you look outside your own environment - to music or dance or social work or teaching or service jobs of all kinds to see people who are making very important contributions. For most reasonable people, it's not hard to be humble in that context. We all have a pretty narrow contribution to make.

That's one piece of it. Then the other piece of it is that, within your own realm, you should set a high goal. Try to do something that matters. Don't waste your time trying to do unimportant things. Make sure that what you're doing is important. Then it's possible to feel good about yourself at the same time that you can see yourself in perspective with other people who are making other kinds of contributions. You can apply that across a pretty broad range. I've worked in a scientific environment, so I often talk to young people about, "Why are you doing this experiment? Why are you doing this study of patients? Is the answer going to be important? Or is it just going to get you another publication?" If the answer is that it will be important, then you should be doing it. If the answer is that it won't be an important contribution but it's a good way to get your next grant, then you need to stop and do something else. I have functioned in various roles in the course of my career, as a scientist, a clinician, a teacher, an administrator, a leader of my professional society. In each of these roles, I was replaceable. We all are, and in the grand scheme of life we will be replaced soon. That's a good thing, but while you have the chance, while you have the time, be sure that you feel you are doing something meaningful.

[Matt: One day when you walk away from medicine and hang up your white coat for the very last time, what do you want to see looking back on medicine?]

I suppose there are two things that matter most to me. The first one is that I would like to look back on my career and know that I had made life a little better for the people I encountered - whether it was patients, co-workers, or students - that there were lives that were better because I had been there. No one can change the life of everyone they encounter, but you'd like to think that you had a positive impact on people' - that their lives were happier, healthier, more successful because of their interaction with you. For me, that's what I want to carry

away at the end - it isn't the tangible accomplishments, the things I tried to build, the research I've done, all of which could be sources of pride. But for me it's very easy - it's about how I've affected the lives of people who depended on me. Given my role in an academic setting, I probably think more about the people I've worked with or taught than I do about patients, although I certainly think about patients as well; it's just that only a relatively small fraction of my time throughout my career has been spent in direct patient care. So that's what I would like to take away when I hang up my coat for the last time - that I helped people have a happier and more fulfilling life.

The second one is probably embarrassing but this interview only has value people are honest: I would like to feel when I walk away from my career that other people appreciate these qualities, think of me kindly, and feel that I've had an impact on their lives.

I'd like to cure cancer too - I say this jokingly because it isn't going to happen. I'd like to have an important contribution in science, but even if I did it would be of less importance to me.

[Matt: To medical students and premedical students in the future, can you share a pearl with us?]

I'm not fond of giving advice, but I've already said maybe two things in different ways that would be the answer to this question. The first is to set yourself a goal that is important, hard, but ultimately achievable, so that you feel you are doing something important. The second is that you get rewarded in life for doing the right thing. It doesn't always feel like that. It sometimes feels like the people who are aggressive or nasty or selfish get their way, and that the people who are kind and generous and thoughtful are pushed aside. I think it's easy for young people to feel that way, and certainly we have all had experiences where we have seen people rewarded for behavior that we don't admire. In the long run in life, there are tangible rewards for being a good human being - not just in terms of your own sense of self, but in terms of the opportunities it creates, in terms of the relationships it facilitates. That's something you only learn with time, that there is a connection between being a good person, doing the right thing, and success.

Dean Ornish

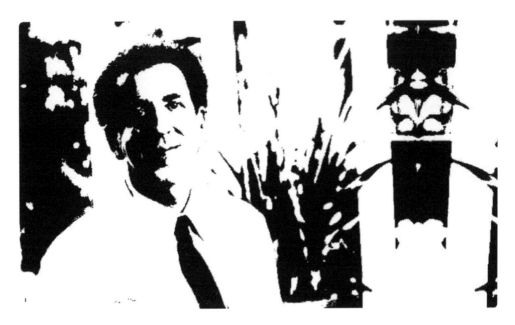

Dean Ornish M.D. is Founder and President of the Preventative Medicine Research Institute, author of six best-selling books including *The Spectrum*, and personal health consultant to President Bill Clinton.

our white coat - The physician's role is to help facilitate healing in the patients by empowering them with information that they can use to make informed and intelligent decisions about their health and well-being. We have found in 36 years of research that our bodies have a re-markable capacity to begin healing themselves

if we simply stop doing what's causing the prob-lem. To a large degree the underlying causes of many, perhaps most, chronic diseases are the lifestyle choices that we make: these include what we eat, how we respond to stress, whether or not we smoke cigarettes, how much exercise we get, and perhaps most important, how much love, intimacy, and community we have in our lives.

In a series of studies over the past 36 years, my colleagues and I at the Nonprofit Pre-ventative Medicine Research Institution, in col-laboration with UCSF and many leading institutions, have found that these lifestyle changes can stop and even reverse the progression of the most common chronic diseases. These include coronary heart disease, early stage prostate cancer, type II diabetes, by extension breast cancer, elevated cholesterol levels, obesity, hypertension, and so on. We found that over 500 genes were changed in just three months, upregulating or turning on the disease-preventing genes and downregulating or turning off the disease-promoting genes.

Our latest study found that these lifestyle changes could lengthen telomeres at the end of our chromosomes; and that any intervention can lengthen telomeres and thus begin to reverse the aging process on a cellular level. We found that the more people change their lifestyle, they more they improve all these different measures. Our work is in educating, empowering, and informing people so they can make and maintain these lifestyle changes, which can therefore aid in their healing process. So both the doctor and the patient are participating in their healing and in the sense are wearing the white coat.

On empowering people to make sustainable changes in their lives - What we've found doesn't work is what most doctors use, which is fear. Fear is not a sustainable motivator, particularly in the area of trying to motivate people to make sustainable changes in lifestyle. In the short run, it's very effective. When someone has had a heart attack, they'll do anything their healthcare professional asks them to do for a month or so, but even then the denial comes back. That's why adherence to statin drugs is only about 30% at 3-4 months, even if someone pays for them and even when they have no side effects, because they're fear based. Take this pill to prevent something really awful like a heart attack or stroke happening years down the road that you don't want to think about. Some people stop thinking about it, so they stop taking it.

Whereas fear of dying is not a sustainable motivator, joy of living is. When people make these changes, most people find that they feel better so much better so quickly, it reframes the reason for making these changes from fear of dying, which is not sustainable, to joy of living, which is. Your chest pain tends to go away, your complexion improves, you can grow brain neurons, your brain can get measurably bigger, your genes can change in just a few months, and so on. There's no point in giving up something you enjoy unless you get something back that makes you feel better, and quickly. Most people find they feel so much better so quickly that these are choices worth making.

The other aspect that's sustainable is a sense of community. We use support groups to help people make these changes, but they're not support groups in the usual sense. It's really creating a safe environment where people feel safe enough to let down their emotional defenses and talk openly about what is going on in their lives without fear that someone is going to judge them. That sense of community is so meaningful that years and sometimes decades after the study ends, people are still meeting together because it's meaningful for them.

It's really the secret sauce that enables us to get 85-90% adherence to a very intensive lifestyle program after a year, whereas adherence to statin drugs is only 30% in three to four months. The idea that taking a pill is easy and everyone will do it, but that changing lifestyle is difficult if not impossible, is really the opposite of what the evidence shows. These biological mechanisms are so dynamic that when we change our lifestyles, we really feel better so quickly that for many people these are choices worth making.

attending to the world - Medicine is all about service. Most of us went into medicine because we wanted to help people. As insipid as that may sound, that's really what drives most physicians. It's not power or money or status, it's service. That's part of the Hippocratic Oath. Unfortunately that desire often gets drummed out of us in the process of our training. But there are some very gifted physicians such as Dr. Naomi Remen and others who are helping people get re-enchanted and reclaim our role as healers that serve rather than technicians or worse, algorithms. If all we were is a collection of algorithms, we'd be replaced by an iPhone app before long because computers can do that better. There's an art of medicine, a service of medicine, as well as a science of medicine, an algorithm of medicine.

When you serve, it empowers you and the person who you're serving. Anything that cre-

ates a sense of connection and community and intimacy is really healing. Even the word "healing" comes from the root "to make whole." The word "yoga" comes from the Sanskrit *yoke*: to unite, to bring together. Study after study has shown that people who are depressed and isolated are more likely to get sick and die prematurely than people who have a sense of love, connection, and community. Service connects us and heals us, both for the doctor and the patient.

Your book itself is a service. After seeing what a powerful difference these simple changes can make, I found my calling. That's what enabled me to spend 16 years in Medicare before they agreed to cover our program. That's why I love doing this work. We tend to think of advances in medicine as being something really high-tech and expensive, a new drug, a new laser, but what we're learning is that these simple ideas like meaning and service are so transformative and powerful not only for these patients but for those who do this work. If it's meaningful, it's sustainable.

uplifting the medically underserved - Access to health is a human right. So much of what we're learning is that the simple choices that we make in our lives each very day are really the primary determinants of our health and well-being. It doesn't necessarily mean access to a physician, though that can be part of it. It's really access to the information and the support that can help people transform their lives for the better, making it easy for people to make the right choices. I worked with McDonalds on putting salads on the menu, and they did that, but the problem was that because of the perverse subsidies on the farm bill, the burger's 99 cents, the salad is $6.95. So if you're on a fixed income, you get a lot more calories for your dollar by eating unhealthy foods, which are the ones that are subsidized because they don't take into account the real costs of the food in terms of the effects on your health and ultimately on medical expenses. How can we create a healthy country? A healthcare system, not a sick-care system, in which we encourage people and support them in making healthier choices, and which would include but not be limited to a physician.

Medicare is now covering our program. They've created a new benefit category called intensive cardiac rehabilitation. We've been training hospitals and clinics around the country. It's a team approach: the doctor's quarterback but there's a nurse, a yoga teacher, an exercise physiologist, a dietician, and a clinical psychologist. Medicare will pay for 72 hours of training at over $100 an hour, which we do in usually 18 four-hour sessions. [Patients] come for an hour of supervised exercise, an hour of stress management, a support group, plus an hour of lecture and a group meal. Once they finish their 72 hours, they continue to meet in a self-directed community. That doesn't require additional expenses, but because the community is so meaningful and powerful, it's a way to sustain the changes and integrate them into their lives on a more permanent basis.

On the role that students can make an impact in medicine and patient care - It's one of the reasons that I spent 16 years working with Medicare before they agreed to cover our program. I used to think if we could do science it would change medical practice. To some degree it did, in the ways we talked about. But reimbursement is a much more powerful determinant of medical practice and even medical education. So I realized that if we could change reimbursement we would change not only medical practice but also even medical education.

We empower students with this information and these experiences. I'm a Clinical Professor of Medicine at UCSF. We have students, house staff, and other disciplines come out and spend time with us. We train and certify them in our program and give them support to continue. Now that Medicare is paying for it, most insurance companies are paying for it as well. Then it becomes standard of care. We're trying to create a new paradigm of healthcare instead of sick care. Now that the Affordable Care Act has survived all the things that were trying to derail it, it turns the incentives on their ear.

Before, the more drugs and surgeries you used, the more money you made as the doctor or surgeon. If you did a bypass or put a stent in, you'd make more money. Now, it's more that there are X dollars to take care of someone, you the doctor gets to keep what isn't spent. The incentives get turned around 180 degrees to programs that are less expensive and more effective. So reducing the economic incentive to operate on people or do procedures that can be done less expensively and more effectively with diet and lifestyle. So there's really a convergence of forces that make this the right idea at the right time. The limitations of high tech medicine have become clear. The randomized trials that were summarized in the Archives of Internal Medicine last year looked at eight randomized trials looked at the stents and angioplasties and find that they don't work, they don't prolong life, they don't prevent heart attacks, they don't reduce angina unless you're in the middle of having a heart attack which most people aren't.

It's not like there's one set of lifestyle interventions for heart disease and a different one for prostate cancer, diabetes, telomere length, or gene expression. It's the same lifestyle interventions for each of these. The more people change, the more they improve. You find similar data for Type II diabetes, which is already pandemic around the world. Yet studies show that lowering your blood sugar with drugs doesn't work nearly as well as lowering it with diet and lifestyle in terms of preventing the complications and cost of Type 2 diabetes. If you get someone's HbA1C down below 7.0 with diet and lifestyle, you can prevent all of these horrible complications of diabetes. Getting the blood sugar down with drugs doesn't necessarily accomplish that goal. The limitations of these high tech approaches are becoming clear, as the same time the power of these low-tech interventions are becoming more well documented, at a time when the reimbursement structure is changing to subsidize less expensive, more effective interventions like the ones we're talking about.

a loving smile - Of course it's appropriate because the doctor-patient relationship is a sacred bond, and it's part of the healing process. You can only be intimate to the degree you can allow yourself to be emotionally vulnerable with someone, only to the degree that you feel a sense trust, and you can only do that to the degree that you feel a sense of a bond and safe. That's why the physician-patient relationship is considered sacred, because that trust is what enables what the physicians recommends to people try, particularly if that involves something painful or dangerous like surgery or medications or something with potentially negative side effects. If you don't trust your doctors, you are less likely to do what you ask them to do. Without trust you have nothing.

My work was ridiculed when I started doing it: "That's a stupid idea, you can't reverse heart disease." If you don't have a sense of meaning and purpose behind it, then it's not sustainable. The fact that people were skeptical and didn't believe it made the work worth doing. That gave me the strength and sense of meaning to persist beyond the obstacles.

a life apart - Authenticity is healing. It's important to express your emotions as feelings rather than thoughts or judgments. So if you said to someone, I feel happy, I feel concerned, I feel angry, I feel upset, I feel depressed- if you can express that as a feeling, it's a gift to the other person. If you use a thought or judgment, if you say, "I think you're wrong, I think you're a jerk, most people are going to react in a negative way. They'll feel attacked and judged and they'll withdraw or attack back. If you give someone an authentic feeling, it's a gift and it'll bring you closer. Since intimacy is healing, then anything that brings us closer together, whether it's with students or patients or spouses or family members or friends, it's moving us in a healing direction.

a story - When I was a second year medical student at Baylor, I was learning to do heart bypass surgery with Michael DeBakey MD, the heart surgeon. It was exciting but also disheartening because we were literally bypassing the problem, we weren't treating the cause. So people would go home and do the things that caused the problem in the first place. More often than not, the bypasses would clog up and we'd cut them open and have to do it three to four times. I started reading the literature to see if there might be a better way. In my first study, I put 10 people in a hotel for a month and put them in this program. It was just me and the chef. We had a 75-year-old dentist who was homophobic and another of the patients was gay. This was Houston in 1977. And the older guy said something really nasty to the younger gay guy, who said something equally awful back. They started yelling at each other. One got chest pain and took a nitroglycerin, one got chest pain and took a Demerol, slammed the door, slammed the door, clutched their chests. I thought, Wow,

they're both going to have heart attacks and die. This is going to be the end of my very short research career.

I talked to both of them separately and said, "Look, you're giving the power of having chest pain and maybe even die from heart attack to the person you're most angry with and maybe even hate. That's not really smart, even for your own self-interest, especially for your own self-interest." I brought them together and said, "The first step in healing is compassion, and love, and service, so I want you guys to spend the next month here." I gave them service tasks to do for each other, doing each other's laundry or whatever. When you forgive somebody, you're more compassionate to someone, it doesn't condone what they've done, but it frees you from the suffering that goes along with that.

It's particularly auspicious to talk about it now, Nelson Mandela just died a few days ago. That's why the whole world was so galvanized behind him. Here's a guy who has every reason to be angry and upset after being in jail for 27 years, but he forgave the people who did that because he knew that in order to accomplish his larger vision of freeing South Africa from apartheid, that he had to let go of his legitimate grievances. Compassion, altruism, and forgiveness are what empower us and free us from our suffering, and free the people around us from their suffering. So to me medicine is more than just algorithms and medications, vital signs, and cholesterol levels, it's really helping people use the experience of suffering as a catalyst for transforming their lives for the better. That really brings us back to a physician as healer rather than simply as a computer or the algorithm.

Dean Schillinger

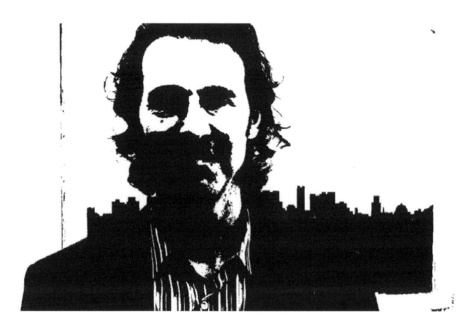

Dean Schillinger M.D. is Chief of the Division of General Internal Medicine at the San Francisco General Hospital and Trauma Center. Dr. Schillinger is also the Director of the Health Communications Program at the UCSF Center for Vulnerable Populations.

our white coat - I work at San Francisco General Hospital and Trauma Center, the public safety net hospital of this city. The white coat, to me and many doctors who take care of patients in underserved settings, is a barrier representing the power imbalance between the privi-

leged health professional- well-trained, well-educated- setting us off as white, starched, and clean, as compared to our patients with lower socioeconomic status. But I think your question is getting at something beyond the white coat. I have an appreciation for what people are going through and the nature of suffering. I understand how feeling is not just a one-time event but is a process and can be incomplete.

I think with an open mind and open heart and try to be mindful of my patient's emotional state as well as the state of their body and spirit. Beyond that, I try to do good doctoring in the traditional sense: take a good history, be obsessive and careful, attempt to make the correct diagnoses, suggest the right decisions and path to take, and motivate the patient to take those paths if I feel they are the right ones. If I don't know which is the right path, I will share in the wisdom of my patient and help her make that decision. I'm appreciative of any progress we can make, and I will be present with them if we're not making progress.

attending to the world - Most physicians, the overwhelming majority of physicians, would steer very clear of these settings. The patients are complex, hard to reach, and don't pay anything. They're felt to be intransigent. So there's a huge unmet need for doctoring in this population. The number of physicians who care for poor patients is inversely proportional to the number for poor patients. By choosing to work here, we choose to serve others.

All healers, all physicians, all clinicians serve others. We just happen to select the underserved to serve, which by its very nature is a quixotic degree of service from a public health standpoint. There's very little I can do as a physician doing the same case over and over and over again to substantively improve the public's health. So we have to do more than take care of the patient one patient at a time. I think many of us choose to serve in other capacities as well: to try to move policy, to try to change the social conditions, to try to reduce health disparities at a higher level.

uplifting the medically underserved - I believe access to a trained health professional, whether it be a nurse practitioner, physician's assistant, or other should be a right in this country definitely. I think my role in pursuing health equity is very multi-dimensional, which is true of many of my doctors who work at my institution. The first is to take outstanding care of a cadre of patients - who are either uninsured, publicly insured, all of whom who have low socioeconomic status, many of whom are minority and come from immigrant populations - to work with them to improve their individual health. Then it's to train the future leaders in the care of the underserved; we run a residency program and medical school. Then it's to do research, to define the nature of health disparities, to get under the skin of health disparities, and try to intervene to mitigate health disparities by generating generalizable knowledge about improvements in care and prevention. Lastly, it's to impact larger policy initiatives to change the social, cultural environments in which health happens or disease happens unequally, and to change that pattern of inequality that leads to health inequities. I've had roles in each of those domains in the course of my career.

a loving smile - The secret to bonding with a patient for me - I have a couple of them. One is of course to elicit their narrative. Tell me your story, tell me who you are, what makes you tick, and what brings you to my office- in a very curious way, because people are very interesting, particularly people we take care of at this hospital [San Francisco General Hospital]. And inevitably, I will find at least one thing that I have in common with that person. The second thing that's very helpful to me in particularly challenging patients is to find one thing that you particularly like about them and say it. The third is to understand their vulnerabilities and their resources and strengths. Once you understand their vulnerabilities you can empathize much more effectively. Once you understand their strengths, you can strategize with them much more effectively. The last thing is the importance of continuity, longitudinal relationships.

a life apart - When is it appropriate to be saddened? I would say whenever something happens that is saddening. It's a basic human emotion. I guess there's sadness and there's depression, so we should distinguish between the two. There are very high rates of depression among physicians, high rates of depressive systems and burn-out among primary care physicians who care for the underserved. I think it's something we need to much more frequently call attention to and see as a target for reductions with respect to how health systems are designed.

With respect to sadness, which I see as more circumstantial, there's plenty to be sad about: people die, limbs get lost, mistakes get made. I think we owe it to ourselves, our colleagues, and to our students to show our humanity and express that sadness. We also try to learn something from the circumstance, try to identify the root causes that led to the event that is leading one to be sad, and then to decide whether or not the sadness is actually shame or guilt or some other unhelpful emotion- or whether it's really a systems problem that needs to be addressed. I think that sharing in the sadness with patients when they have a bad diagnosis or bad outcome is our shared humanity.

a story - I will just say to look at the poem by Marge Piercy, entitled "To Be of Use." It really beautifully conveys the importance of being that person in a fireline who's passing the water pail down the line and how important that person is as opposed to the parlor general who's calling the shots. "To Be of Use" is my inspirational poem for a first-year medical student.

a lens into your life - I'd say, having very bad things happen to my family over the course of their history led me to feel some belief in justice, that there needs to be justice. My uncle was very influential to me. He ran UNESCO's education program for science to teach the developing world about science, so I think I gained an interest in public health through that. But my residency training was very formative for me. And it was during that residency training that I had the pleasure of working in a public hospital. Most states and cities don't have public hospitals anymore. They tore them down in the 60s and 70s because they lose money. Some of the medical schools still have public hospitals and some don't.

I came to train at UCSF, which has San Francisco General Hospital. I came here with a lot of biases. I was scared. It was the AIDS epidemic. But working here was transformative because you saw very bright people working on an epidemic that was devastating. Young men were dying left and right. We and they took an approach that was mindful of the clinical concerns, engaged the public health department and society at large, as well as the scientific community, to, within a generation, basically solve an epidemic. That was a very inspiring environment to be in. I wasn't aware of how it was shaping me at the time; it probably is still shaping me. When you have a stigmatized disease with stigmatized patients in a stigmatized hospital, and yet you're going into that room 5-6 times a day with all of your heart and all of your mind, to do the best you can as difficult as it is, because other people are modeling it for you, it becomes a way of life. You begin to feel the higher meaning of it, in ways that go beyond doing that in a private hospital. There's something more when it's someone who is otherwise powerless and meaningless to society. It's pretty amazing.

The other part of it was becoming a primary care physician here. The face of public hospitals are the patients who come to our clinics. Being a primary care doctor here for 20 years has really motivated me because I feel like I really understand people in a different way than when you're an inpatient doctor taking care of someone for four days. Being connected to someone who lives in a community, who comes from a family, who has barriers, obstacles, challenges, strengths, resources, who values what we bring to them as an institution, just reinforces it. 5A was the AIDS ward when I was a resident and trainee: door-to-door HIV, dying men with HIV. If you walk in there now, it's all diabetes. People get amputations, kidney failure with diabetes. It's just a different epidemic now. Being a practitioner allows one to observe what's going on in society and try to respond to it. I think you have to stay engaged in practice.

Ellen Beck

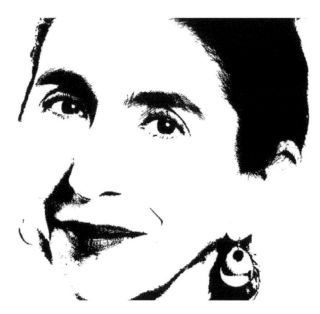

Ellen Beck, M.D. is Clinical Professor and Founding Director, with passionate students and outstanding community partners, of the University of California, San Diego (UCSD) Student Run Free Clinic Project.

our white coat - Our work is to empower: to create environments where the other, individual, family, and community can take charge of their lives and achieve joy and well-being.

attending to the world - The community is our teacher: the community, the patient, will teach us how to be an effective physician to them. We must always be aware of not only the patients we serve, but all of those who cannot get in the door. We need not only to provide care to all, but that care

must be a type of health care that is respectful, thorough, and addresses social determinants of health. It saddens me that a country as wealthy as ours has not matured to realize that health care is a right. I often teach my students, to paraphrase Buehner, that there are infinite needs in the world, to find one of their great passions and match it to that need. Martin Luther King, Jr. taught "Injustice anywhere is a threat to justice everywhere." There are so many injustices, locally and globally. Find one about which you are passionate and do something to address it.

a loving smile - A humanistic approach means to imbue each interaction, as Carl Rogers taught, with respect, empathy, and self-awareness. We must build bridges of trust to our patients and help them address their fears. I add two questions to my history - to ask patients not only their sources of stress, but also their sources of strength. The first prescription that I teach students to write is a 'sources of strength' prescription for their patients. Also, being able to smile is important to our health and our self worth. As part of our trans-disciplinary model, I teach that 'toothlessness leads to joblessness.'

a life apart - I teach our students that when a tear comes, they are Las Jollas de Amor, that we are touching love or truth.

a story - When we first saw one of our elderly patients at the free clinic project, she was so gaunt and disabled that we saw her in her family's car because it was too painful and difficult for her to get out. Now she has been our patient or 15 years. As she became more and more functional and happier, she began to gain weight, and now we follow her for diabetes. A medical student involved in her care at the free clinic project recently said, Mrs. S. was my first continuity patient. They have showed me that the reason I got into medicine is out there, the people that I want to help, the people I want to come alongside. This is the experience I want for the rest of my life."

The doctors who now supervise her treatment were medical students when they were first involved in her care. Recently, we were her guests at her granddaughter's quinceañera. This year we gave her adult daughter an Angel award at our yearly gala for taking such diligent loving care of her mother, for being her advocate, and for making it possible for her mother to experience joy and well-being.

a lens - When I was young, I faced a number of life challenges. My half-brother committed suicide when I was five years old, and my half-sister developed a psychosis and remained that way for the rest of her life. I assumed that my life would probably end in suicide or mental illness, just like my brother and sister. In my mid-20's, I realized that no matter what bad things had happened, I could paint the picture of my life, I could be the artist of my existence. Once I learned this for myself, I wanted to create environments where I could do the same for others. It is a tremendous honor to be seen as someone who inspires others. That gift demands humility and that I do my best to become the person others see. I have started now to see who other people see when they look at me, and every day I work on becoming that person.

uplifting the underserved - This phrase is not one I would use. If anything, the underserved uplift us and can be our life teachers, about facing challenges, about overcoming obstacles, about knowing that which is truly important. They inspire and 'uplift' me daily. Implicit in the word underserved, is that we as a society are underserving large segments of our society. Implicit in the word is that there is a right to health care. When we think even for a moment we are uplifting the underserved, it is as if in some way we are above them but, no, we are all human beings together. We can empower, that is, create environments where people take charge of their lives, but the word uplifting unintentionally can make it seem that we are better, higher, it seems almost paternalistic. Also, the word uplifting can have religious connotations. We must never proselytize, we must never try to convince someone else to follow our beliefs or faith. Our role is to help people identify their sources of strength and to encourage them to integrate these into their lives.

Fabien Koskas

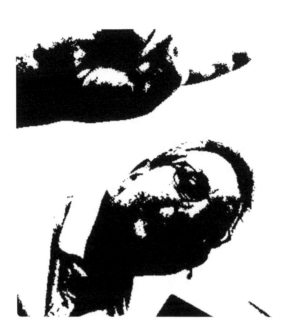

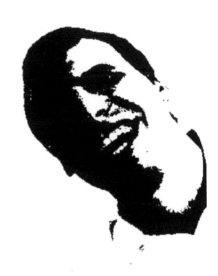

Fabien Koskas, M.D. is a Chief of Vascular Surgery at Pitié-Salpêtrière University Hospital in Paris, France.

attending to the world - It's a service. It's different from general practice scenarios. It's life saving or life preserving. This is the way it is different. You never have to do that, generally the patient is sleeping (smile). It is extremely difficult. You try not being impressed at the general attitude of the patient. One way of doing this is to focus on the disease and not the patient. Diseases pertain to particular patients. You have to adapt between two extremes. You have the life of a patient in the palm of your hands. You have a critical mission you have to accomplish one way or another. There is no way outside of this way. Our field is seeing people getting better and better. This is our main field. It's not money, it's not personal success. It is to see the patients we have in charge, improve.

Isaac Yang

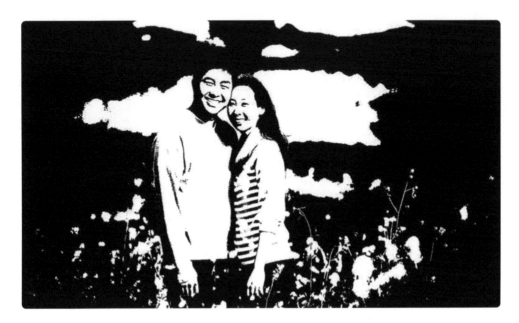

Isaac Yang, M.D. is Assistant Professor of Neurosurgery at the David Geffen School of Medicine at the University of California, Los Angeles.

our white coat - I think of my white coat as a superman's cape, not so much because I'm Superman, but because of the way patients see me in my white coat. It tells them, 'He's going to do the right thing,' it's my cape.

attending to the world - I went to UC Berkeley for my bachelor's degree, UCLA for medical school, UCSF for residency, and now I'm on the faculty at UCLA Medical School. I have no right to turn down anyone. I'm indebted to the people of California. I don't ask if my patients have insurance, I ask if they have a brain tumor.

a loving smile - My name Isaac means 'to smile' or 'to laugh.' Laughter is the best medicine. Sometimes we can't help our patients. We haven't found the cure for brain cancer yet, but we can always hold a hand and give a hug. We can always make our patients feel better.

a life apart - You can always feel sad. I let myself feel both happy and sad, the important thing is not to let our emotions interfere with the care of our patients. We can use every experience, whether good or bad, happy or sad, to become a better doctor.

a lens - We are all human, everyone has someone important to them, close loved ones. For me, it's my wife. When I see a patient I see them as someone else's loved one, and think if they were my loved one, I would want to do everything I possibly could to do the right thing for her {photo is of Dr. Yang and his wife, Nancy Yang}.

Josh Broder

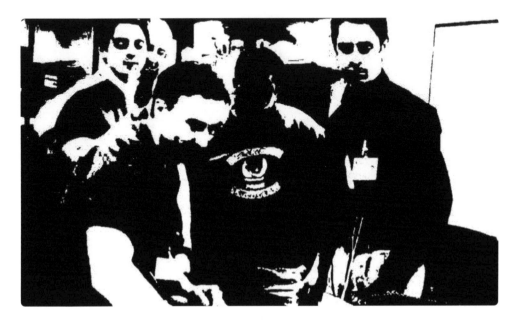

Josh Broder M.D. is Associate Professor of Surgery, Division of Emergency Medicine at Duke University School of Medicine, and serves as the Duke University Emergency Medicine Residency Program Director.

our white coat - I don't usually wear a white coat when I'm working. I tend to be on my knees helping the nurses, residents, and medical students down in the trenches—in the trauma bays. I'm not sure wearing a white coat is a practical model in the emergency department. Yet, it is an interesting idea that the white coat is a symbol of the doctor-patient relationship. It can be valuable and it can remind physicians that they have a responsibility to the patient. Nonetheless, sometimes the white coat can be too hierarchical. It can create a hierarchy where the patient is expected to accept what the physician has to say without challenge. People have white coat hypertension for a reason. Though we must not forget, the white coat can sometimes also be a vehicle for communication. Studies suggest that patients see the white coat as a surrogate for knowledge. If you have never seen a particular physician before, when it is an emergency, you know you can trust that person on first sight as a result of the white coat. Thus, I see some potential value.

On the topic of the patient-doctor relationship, I often think that the relationship should be reversed a little bit. If you believe in the concept of the physician as a public servant, we belong to the patient. They are not ours, we are theirs. Their decisions about their own healthcare are decisions for them to make, instead of us dictating to the patient. If the patient is "my patient," it suggests an ownership relationship in which I could do with the patient what I want. It is extremely important to remember that no one belongs to us - if anything, we belong to them. But I think that the relationship should not be one of ownership on either end, and instead be mutual. In order for it to be a therapeutic relationship, there must be feelings of mutual investment. Investing yourself in the patient, you want to promote a sense of belonging, a sense of empowerment. When a patient is empowered, they have the authority to say to the physician, "Tell me more or give me choices about what we are supposed to do for my health." This will be most rewarding to you as a physician in return.

attending to the world - I have spent a little over a decade now as an attending physician, and my role has shifted over time. As a resident physician, you are very much attending to the patient directly. You get to ask questions, order tests, and figure out what the patient will do when they go home. The attending physician is an academic physician, in a more supervisory role, and so my time at the bedside has been shortened. As a result, I have come to value my time with my patients. I value time with the residents and students too. I feel fortunate to have a lot of different directions within which to work. At the end of the shift, I often ask my self, "Did I do a good job, did I teach people, did I teach patients things? Did I give good medical care??" It is really not just a job, because patients physiologically and psychologically rely on you, and there is a burden of responsibility to perform at an extremely high level of service at all times. Baseball players are exceptional when they bat .500. We as physicians have to serve and get the job right 100% of the time if we want patient outcomes to be good. I don't always come away from my shift feeling like I met the challenge. I come home very tired, and say I am going to work on this tomorrow and become a better physician. There are times we forget what the over-riding purpose is. You have to remember why you went into medicine. Most people are very driven by the notion of service, and medical students applying to our residency program have statements that revolve around serving other people. We worry that the process of training physicians undermines empathy. It is the responsibility of the attending physician not to appear jaded. We are role modeling for developing resident physicians and they embody everything that we do. If you don't go into rooms with residents, and discuss cases after the resident sees the patient, you don't get the opportunity to model for the resident what service means. Even something simple such as asking if the patient what they feel and what they are worried about. I think that being a physician is inherently a complex role. Serving other people is inherently an altruistic pursuit, yet also self-serving at the same time. You have to take care of yourself if are going to give service to others and avoid burnout. You have to find satisfaction. There are rewards inherently in feeling you have done a good job for other people. You may have a certain sense of renewal in that process. It is part of being human, and gives you the energy to return.

uplifting the medically underserved - Emergency medicine is really a field that is rooted in that concept of universal service and universal care. We have a federal mandate, and the vast majority of emergency physicians don't feel that it is an imposition on the field that everyone who comes to the emergency room in the United States deserves a screening medical exam even without the ability to pay. It is a wonderful legal protection. We must ask why they are there and what they need from us. I certainly am a big supporter of universal access to healthcare. Does that mean every single medical service should be available to all people? It is hard to know because there is the question of societal resources which can be brought up. If you allocate all services to one patient, should that compromise service to others? In a completely unconstrained system, you would supply everything to everyone. It is a very complex question. I think that it is a key role for physi-

cians, emergency medicine physicians specifically, to ensure that all of our patients have care. As an example, there are some states, that are looking at legislation that would second-guess the right to care in the emergency department. Tremendous cost would have to be borne upon many of their patients' shoulders, and might discourage people from pursuing that care. We have to use a lay-person definition of an emergency. We can't expect every person to have medical expertise. Instead, for a reasonable person, the question must simply be, is it something serious? We should respect patients' perspectives; it is not appropriate to look back on people's care. So the right to be seen and cared for must be preserved, and not be barriers to people's lives.

We must not forget that there are barriers that exist because of socioeconomic status. If you don't have transportation or if there is a copay, you are not going to seek care until you are sicker than you would otherwise be. Preventative medicine is in the patient's interest and in society's interest. The cost of end of life care and critical care are much higher than prevention. That is the pragmatic reason, not the ethical reason.

Sometimes we may not approve of the way in which a colleague speaks to a patient because of their race, socioeconomic status, cultural background, or even at a repeat visit. A person may want to be a good physician, want to free themselves of prejudice and say to others, "The way that you treated the patient made me uncomfortable," but the moment of confrontation is difficult. If they have the right values they will probably thank you for it, because the goal isn't to create shame. Yet, if you do it in private (to protect the person from shame), what is the message to students and trainees? What about other physicians and co-workers? You will have to go back and do it twice. You have to emphasize to your team not to forget about the patient in the process, and there are times you probably owe it to the patient to say something to them too. In a perfect world, everyone would recognize the misdeed, maybe even get the particular personnel to come back and speak to the patient themselves. Together, we are working toward a better profession.

a loving smile - It is totally appropriate to show emotion in front of trainees. It is not harmful to show emotion in front of the patient. When I see a really sad outcome, a patient death, I actually end up connecting with the family and the other loved ones more than the patients themselves. If the patient comes in awake and alive, then my emotions are more attracted to them. In emergency medicine, it is not uncommon for patients to come in after death. If it is a grandchild, son or daughter in the waiting room, my sadness and sympathy will be extended to them. I'm not going to stop myself from trying to comfort them. It is quite common in my practice for me to hug a relative and not uncommon for me to cry with the residents and nurses, as well as in a family's room. If you can spend just a moment with a patient or a patient's family, displaying the human touch and saying, "I'm

really sorry about what has happened and genuinely feel what you are feeling," then these aren't crocodile tears. When I have a genuine sense of sadness, it actually lets me get back to the rest of my responsibilities really quickly. A big part of medicine is understanding that death is a natural part of life. Not all deaths make me sad. The losses make me sad. When I was in residency, I lost my grandparents. I remember how that felt and those memories flash back when I am interacting with a family that has experienced a great loss. And I think I can learn from that experience.

Today I worked in the pediatric emergency room. I treated a teenager in the pediatric ICU, who had many near death experiences. Her mother was very scared. As a resident, I was often under the impression that I wasn't supposed to react or acknowledge what another person is going through. Today, first thing I did was I took this woman's hand and just gave her a hug and said we are going to do everything we can, and she smiled. She knew she could trust us. It is about figuring out an appropriate boundary. I definitely would encourage physicians to not be afraid to show genuine emotion; it is not a weakness, and it is not a lack of professionalism.

At the same time sometimes we take ourselves too seriously in medicine. There is an ophthalmologist in Florida who uses blow up dolls to illustrate principles, and when I saw him I learned so much in 20 minutes of watching him. In some ways, I think laughter trains your brain to retain information. It is ok to make a joke and engage in laughter.

Linda Regan

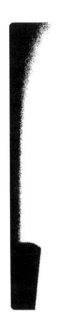

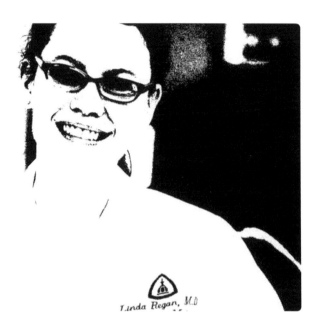

Linda Regan M.D. is Residency Program Director at the Johns Hopkins Emergency Medicine Residency Program.

our white coat - The white coat I think is interesting. I have thought about it quite a bit, the white coat has been traditionally seen as the role of healer. In a traditional sense, it used to represent this aura of respect. But today, I think it more so represents a shared bond between doctor and patient. I personally like to think about the white coat as representing a couple of things. It shows that I care enough about my patients to dress professionally around them. When you ask many patients what makes a physician, a white coat is on many of their lists. People are more likely to pick physicians who are wearing white coats than those who are not wearing them. The white coat highlights the core values that patients see their doctors having, and which their doctors need to uphold. I also like to think that it represents my ability to see my patients for who they are, in the purist sense. When I have my white coat on, no ones' background matters; we are all just people working together to get someone well. I will say that it can create a hierarchical boundary, but I do my best to not view it as such.

To wear a white coat represents to my patients that they should trust me. It does instill that in the patient, it leads patients to say, "this is my physician; this is someone whom I can rest my life in their hands."

attending to the world - As an educator, being an attending means teaching other people to serve as well. I really get to be an attending to the world, as anyone can walk through the door, and there is no distinction between any of our patients. It doesn't matter what you did before the moment I meet you. Every patient is treated the same. That is a challenge, though, as an educator, sometimes you need to teach other physicians how to recognize their own bias, and how to overcome that. That can be challenging at times. If you don't have recognition or insight into yourself and your own struggles, you can't really understand how to best serve your patients, and you can't really understand how to best serve yourself either. Those biases get in the way of being the person who can treat everyone. We can treat people from the moment before they are born to the moment they die, at every stage of their life, no matter what they have been through or what is to come. It is really a phenomenal job that I am tremendously lucky to be doing. I get to help other people learn that they can do better than they often think they can do.

uplifting the medically underserved - You probably could speak to lots of physicians from various specialties; the more uniform answer from doctors in the ED is that there is no place where disparities are more obvious than the emergency department. Many years ago, patients could be turned away if they didn't have money or insurance, now there are laws that require them to treat you, no one can be turned away. I guess emergency departments are really the front door of the hospital. They are used frequently by people who have no other place to go. Helping people who are in your beds and when your beds are full, even in the waiting room. I often view my "office" as the place where I get to take care of everyone, regardless of whether anyone else chooses to treat them. Emergency medicine is the field where we recognize that we are a final, common pathway for everyone to be seen. It can be a challenge, yet I think it is a blessing that you get to be there for these patients.

a loving smile - Patients need to see that you are a normal person. In particular, where I work, I need my patients to trust me immediately. I need them to feel like they can tell me anything about their lives. Looking at the patient like you are there for them, like you are totally focused on them in that moment, smiling doesn't mean you are having a great time, it means you are open and receptive to that person. You are bonding with their experience, and you are understanding their experience. Patients are never going to discuss their lives with the full truth, or fill that prescription if they don't think you are there for them. I do think the ability for patients to see you as someone who has an interest in them, and who views them as important is key. You want them to know that you are not someone who is just going to tell them what to do, but that you are going to integrate their view—that's good care. You want them to think to themselves, "I can't fail, I trust and I'm working with a doctor."

a life apart - I think physicians struggle with the challenge of having empathy or sympathy with their patients. The hardest experience is when you can truly empathize with a person whether it is the loss of a parent or child, or family member they held dear to them. There is actually a debate amongst physicians over whether we should share parts of our lives with patients, whether or not we should choose to share the details about our personal experiences. But I've always thought that patients understand caring; they can sense sadness and compassion in your body, in your words. How you choose to talk with them, the honesty of tears you may have for their loss. Expressing and sharing sadness with patients and their families reminds them that you see them or their loved one not just as a patient, but as a person. It is important for trainees to see that you don't lose that part of yourself in medicine. The moment I no longer care or am affected by what I do and see, is the moment I should stop practicing. I think that it is hard, you have to learn to compartmentalize those pieces, so you can walk out

of one room and walk into another room with a smile on your face. Role modeling that is extremely important for trainees. I have gone home and sat in my car and cried outside my house to avoid being upset in front of my kids. And knowing that I allow my patients to see that I am affected by them and their struggles is the only way I can feel I am giving them everything. I found out that when I share personal details about my own life, they know that I cared for them as a person and not just as a patient. There are boundaries to this, and I avoid sharing things about my kids, but it is important that our trainees know they can do this too.

a story - I had a patient about five years ago, who had been waiting a very long time to see a doctor. She had even brought her suitcase in with her. When an ED physician sees a patient with a suitcase, this normally means the patient thinks that they are going to be admitted, often when they actually don't need to. I volunteered to go and see this patient, who was not on my team, as the physician who was primarily supposed to see her seemed to be having a bad day and I had the feeling this patient might be challenging to them. This woman was pretty angry that she had been waiting a long time. The moment I walked in, to her room, she was angry at me. She raised her voice and started yelling. I just sat down next to her and listened. She had chronic back pain, she had been waiting weeks for an appointment. She didn't understand that her pain would take a while to go away and that taking the medication only when she had pain was not the correct approach. No one had ever explained her medical problem to her and what was actually being done to manage it. She had no idea what to expect about the course of her disease. She didn't feel like a part of her care, and as a result, she was not taking the medicines that had been prescribed. She needed help navigating the clinic system, and she needed someone to explain things to her. When we were done, she said "thank you, that was the most helpful interaction I have ever had." I told her I would email the doctor she was supposed to see. If they could move up her appointment, I would let her know right away. When I was walking her out, there was another patient in a bed in the hallway, who was equally upset over her wait. This patient stopped and walked me over to this new patient in the hall, and she said, "I don't know how long you have been waiting, but if this is the doctor you are waiting to see, she is completely worth the wait." It struck me that from the perspective of "medicine" I hadn't really done anything for this woman, didn't give her any medicine, and didn't offer her anything other than my time and the ability for her to understand her health. It was sad to me that this is probably not uncommon in medicine. We forget that doctors just need to listen to people and explain things to them. Sometimes I think that patients just want you to talk to them and want you to listen to them and their sadness and understand why they are there. I tell my residents to remember that every time you talk to a patient. They might think that she wouldn't be happy unless

she got admitted, but she really needed something else entirely: time and patience.

a lens into your life - I really feel content being with patients and teaching residents how to be better at what they do. That is not just knowledge. That's the entire experience of being a healer. Sometimes, it is just about being a good person.

Lloyd Michener

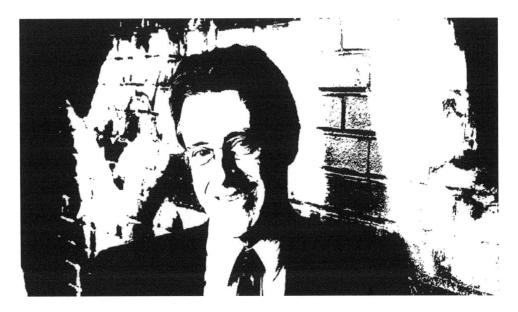

Lloyd Michener M.D. is Chairman of the Department of Community and Family Medicine at Duke University School of Medicine.

our white coat - While training as a medical student at Harvard, I worked in underserved communities where the white coat was often off-putting, especially in community settings. As an intern at Duke, I would wear my white coat, but not a tie. This led to an interesting discussion with one of our senior attendings about appropriate attire. Dr. Eugene Stead commented that we dress in order to make our patients feel comfortable, not to make ourselves feel comfortable. He continued by explaining that the white coat, while it can be seen as a way of distancing ourselves from our patients, can also be seen as a way of a way of communicating safety and security – and that wearing a tie represents that we are bringing our most professional side to each appointment. Ever since then I've worn a white coat and tie during patient care as a sign that my patients and I are together in shared space and time, and that I am in their service. But when I go to community meetings, I don't wear a white coat because I'm there as a member of the community.

attending to the world - I consider medicine a calling. Being a physician invokes very deep beliefs about why we're here and what we're called to do. It's trying to understand the life journey of another individual, knowing that he or she is very different from oneself, and trying to find achievable ways to help. It's about service to the person we're with first, and also to their family, their loved ones, and their community. My goal is to help these people achieve their life goals.

I work as a family doctor within underserved communities. Many of our day-to-day problems are conditions we know how to prevent. So, we work with the communities to help them find the different ways to prevent disease, in addition to helping individuals who are suffering. One of the big projects we're working on at the Center of Community Research is trying to understand why rates of heart disease, cancer, and obesity are so high in some of our underserved communities. If you try to control for the effect of education and income, the differences persist, and we're trying to find out why. For example, our community looked at local grocery store data and obesity rates. From the data came the decision to change zoning laws as well as to get a tax abatement that would attract a grocery store that offers fresh fruits and vegetables to areas with high rates of obesity. The grocery store is under construction now. We didn't do it, but we worked with the community to help them find this solution to a widespread problem.

uplifting the medically underserved - Access to health care services is an essential right. Sometimes it may be a doctor, a nurse practitioner, or a dietitian, but it's always someone who can help the patient with his or her problems. In the U.S. we often think of a doctor, but I work a lot in other countries, and doctors as we know them are not universal. Access to health care is part of equity - one of the fundamental ethical principles. As I look at our communities I see vast disparities in how long people live and the complication rates of diabetes or stroke. It's not tenable to simply observe those differences or to just tell people to seek care. We have to figure out why the differences are so great and how to decrease them. What's striking to me is that you can make a difference. It's hard to make disparities of this magnitude go away completely - though I'm committed to doing that - but we can make a difference in the appalling disparities across ethnicity, race, and gender. I think that's a place in which medical students have a key role. Students looking at disparities can come up with solutions that more senior physicians may miss. For instance, we have a large Latino community in Durham, and our young researchers are working with this community to develop an app that encourages school children to exercise more. For me this is a great example of tailoring solutions to speak to the unique interests and needs of different populations.

a loving smile - It's hard to think of a patient who I don't have some bond with. Whether it's a hallucinating schizophrenic or an alcoholic who's homeless, or a professor, you're always dealing with human beings. If you don't have the emotional sense of bonding, then you belong somewhere else. The necessary part of healing is establishing that bond. It takes seconds. When you go into a room with a person, it's the ability to create that spark of connection that allows us to help others heal. I can't think of a case when it'd be inappropriate to bond.

But there is a balance. After years of bonding with your patients, you can get worn out. It's emotionally tough. That's part of what I like about being a family doc; I always get to see new folks with different issues, so there's the joy of the new and there's also the letting go. There are times when you have to separate emotion and professionalism so that you can tell people things they don't want to hear or deal with. One of the patients I cared for early in the AIDS epidemic was a pastor who had unprotected sex with another man. He was struggling to deal with that as well as whether or not he was going to talk to his wife. That was a case where there was bonding, but there was also a moral obligation, if not a legal one, to his wife. He did what he needed to do, but he had to find his own path, fairly quickly. He died a few years later.

I'm now taking care of third generations, and increasingly find that my role isn't to tell people what to do. I don't find that to be very effective. Rather, my role is to listen, to connect, and to find ways in which I can help. It doesn't take very long to develop that sort of relationship, but it does take some work to become skilled at it. This is where, as you go through medical school, having people record you with individuals and families is incredibly useful. When I went through training, we repeatedly practiced meeting and listening to patients. You may think you're behaving in a way you're not. These practice session helped us overcome this barrier. It's a learnable skill that makes you effective.

a life apart - I worry about physicians who don't feel sadness and joy, because they're taking care of people for whom there are moments of great joy and moments of great sadness. Being with your patients includes sharing these emotions, even if there is nothing you can do but bear witness. Being a healer involves being with your patients through those ups and downs, and helping them make the choices that respect their needs, values and desires. One of the noblest moments I've ever felt was during a home visit with an elderly black woman who was dying at her home with her kids, grandkids, and great-grandkids surrounding her. She was passing with a sense of achieving her life's work. This loss was also one of the most profound, moving, joyous moments I've had, and it was a privilege to be there.

a story - Telling people to exercise more is not reasonable if there are no sidewalks or safe places for them to exercise. Helping neighborhoods become safer is part of a physician's role.

It's been really fun to work with our students in supporting communities - not by lecturing to members of the community - but by helping them find solutions that work for their unique community. It's fun because the communities and students get enthusiastic and come up with things we've never thought about.

For example, there is a group of churches that we work with, and we received a little bit of money to support diet and exercise in their communities. We asked the pastors what they wanted to do. They said what would really help them is if they could have a couple of pairs of running shoes. They held competitions to see who could walk the most in their congregations, and whoever walked the most in a month received a new pair of running shoes. It encouraged the whole group to exercise more.

Another learning experience is related to conducting home visits at our local housing projects. We've come to learn that when there's a gang around your car, it's not necessarily a bad sign. Sometimes these groups know what you're doing and want to watch out for you and your car.

a lens into your life - There is a photo of me in a graffiti-covered school hallway. It's inspiring to me because it says that medicine isn't just about doctors or clinics, it's about embedding health care and access to health care in the community. The photograph was taken at one of the schools we're working with to create a community health hub. *(Editor's Note: This image is featured on Dr. Michener's cover page).*

Louise Aronson

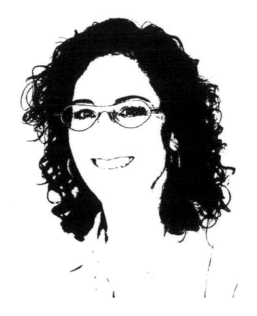

Louise Aronson M.D. is author of *A History of the Present Illness* and Professor of Geriatrics at UCSF Medical Center.

our white coat - I actually don't own a white coat. One of the reasons for that is that I do feel like it can be a divider. It says, I am in this role; it almost puts the role before the humanity of the physician. Saying this is something that identifies me as a doctor means when you look down a hallway, you see doctor instead of person. Moreover, white coats can collect a lot of germs. For me there also is a practical level to not wearing one. At this point in my life, I do mostly house calls. It would be inappropriate and dangerous for me to be walking around in a white coat, yet for me it is more philosophical than that. I think I can be a doctor and a human being at the same time. I feel like that is something I can communicate by how I practice. In not wearing a white coat, I try to break down those barriers between doctor and my patients. We are merely two people who both bring important skills to these encounters. They know themselves better than I, such as their financial status, family relations, daily activities, and I do know the medicine better than they do. It is a collaborative process with people working together to get good medical care, and ultimately better health.

attending to the world - I think if you're attending, whether you are or aren't in an academic context, you are attending to many things simultaneously. You are attending to the patient, and the care of the patient. You need to attend to the caregivers, attend to the education environments and the nurses. You are shepherding the next generation of physicians, so you're promoting their independence and their learning, trying to support their development. Through the patient care and through the teaching, it is just inherent in the role that it is about taking care of those things that only get their significance through the human beings involved in them, whether they are the students, the residents, the patients, or the family. It is not that doctors who are attending only to patients' machinery (an organ, a disease) aren't attending, but we just can't only learn about disease and organ systems. People are human beings. How does that come into play in an individual's life? I don't see how you can divorce organ systems and being human. I am disappointed in the many people who are not appreciating such systems as a human being.

We can often call patients non-compliant and difficult; yet, it is when we are paying too much attention to disease and organ systems and not enough to the human being. If you could pay more attention to what is important to the human being, people would be healthier and have improved outcomes, and in turn you would improve the human condition.

uplifting the medically underserved - I absolutely believe health care is a fundamental human right. I feel like there is this hypocrisy in which people accept that there is a universal right to a fire department, police, and education; yet we want to deprive some people of healthcare, as if those things don't all go hand in hand. All of these settings are essential to society. Even if your only concern were money, it just doesn't make for a good strategy. If your concern is other people and having an optimal functional population, I really think that you need universal healthcare. I think the essential first step is universal access. If you think of marginalized or vulnerable populations, every week more articles show how people of different backgrounds and different ethnicities probably don't all have equal care. This includes everything from the biological level on up; there was another study this week about Vitamin D metabolism measurement and disparate outcomes when the disease is the same. This is a core focus in my life and in my work. One of the primary goals of my book is to humanize people to help people recognize our diversity and also our commonality. The idea was to tell many different stories about many different types of people. When people don't see people as one and other, they can very easily turn off their sense of self. They start to see people as a status or category, and not as a person. When people see them as a category, they can easily deny them health care. Yet when they respond as people, they see the issue as the same as for their kid and respond in the same way that they would as a parent. Of course they will care about their child or aging relative, and the more we can feel, the better. What I have done in my career is see how we tell stories about medicine and about health care, ascribing people status instead of common humanity. It is exciting to reconsider this, interesting, and extremely medically relevant. In medical school, students are often inclined to pursue specialties given different pushbacks, the dumb luck of rotation X, and seeing people do this. It is important, no matter what specialty you choose, to pursue people.

a loving smile - I think bonding with patients is one of the best things about being a doctor. It almost echoes the white coat thing, what I want between me and them. I think people often say history is 70 or 80 percent of the diagnosis. One's ability to get the right history and understand the importance depends upon the relationship. That's why I have done outpatient care in a variety of settings. People are what matter most. You can make a huge difference for someone with personal care and travel to the community that they are in. I want to emphasize that with dying people, you want to teach and maintain dignity and comfort. I really treasure my patient relationships, so I really care about my patients; I think they know that it is with love and affection, almost without exception. You very rarely can't find some shared kernel of human-

ity. For someone in pain who is going through something difficult, if you can give them that loving smile, you usually get one back, and people feel better. I think you need boundaries to do your job and be in your role, but I don't think those things preclude intimacy and affection. This just opens the door for people to give you the accurate history, the relevant history. The history is the story. The history shows you are interested. Really listening so that you help them also humanizes them. I think I am very much a human being with my patients, and it seems to work from both sides.

I understand that some surgeons might feel a little differently on this. Whatever you do, hopefully you love the creativity and precision. You better be enjoying the process itself and not just the outcome. Really think about how you'd like to spend your time. If you are highly technical, the more that you do, the better you will get. Do it because you love it; otherwise do something else. When I was a resident, we worked more than the 70 hours per week maximum that residents have today. I learned that it's not so much about the time, but about using the time in the right way. And just know, at least from years at the Internal Medicine window of the world, you can find secondary gain in working a lot. Your efforts become more precise. And ultimately, I would like to acknowledge you for the amazingly precise work that you do.

It is not always a happy ending to have more time and work less hard. The work hours restrictions on residents have actually made residents less happy, according to many studies.

When we worked 90-100 hours every week, we ate, showered, slept, and didn't really have to make too many other life decisions. Every three to four days we could go out and do something. We lived a pretty simple, straightforward life. You essentially lived at the hospital and in your impromptu exhaustion were there as a whole person. There was never the "Ugh, I'm not working, this or that, should I go hang out with them?" It was likely a false comfort, but you didn't even have to make any decision or prioritize. Busyness can really protect people from a lot of things. As a doctor you will be a certain amount of busyness and your free time might become a crutch. Working a lot can make you feel at one with the profession.

a life apart - What would scare me probably more than any other attribute is, how will you care for others if you have lost a connection to them? We can't be swayed only by sad things; I think that this is inherent. It's sad because you are doing work that is important and meaningful. Those losses and what is at stake are the trade-off in the meaningfulness of the work. To feel safe requires learning how to manage these matters. I think it is essential to show emotion, showing you are sad or anything else. If we don't model that it is actually appropriate to be human, natural, professional, to feel sad when something really sad happens, we are sending this message that to be a doctor is inhumane. Most people can't do it. Most find a place in medicine where that is more or less the standard, the not feeling or not showing feel-

ings. Yet, there are enough data to suggest that when it is, for most people, it comes at a tremendous cost. Physicians have the highest rate of suicide, substance abuse, and divorces. They carry a lot that needs to be dealt with responsibly, professionally, continually. The more we engage sincerely, the healthier we will be and better able to do our jobs.

a story - Anybody who gets up and who doesn't do medicine just for money, to drive a sports car, is a hero. It is interesting to me to see a lot of my friends, who have different roles, do the things that they do. I feel like there is something so special [about medicine] in that it is totally about people; because you can have intimate interactions with people of all types and really intellectual pursuits that range from science to sociology. I go into the projects, into a neighborhood where most everyone does not look like me. I am a geriatrician, so I am going to see an older family member. People were looking out for me and looking out for my car. It's something about us giving. You get something back. Either people are horrified or they say oh my gosh, that's so good. I feel like there are those little moments that they and you can and should be aware of as defining a physician. The benefits to you as a person are so much more and meaningful than some of the things that are distracting people now.

I was as a kid always interested in books and in people. I actually picked an undergraduate college based on its not having any math or science requirements. A doctor was not something I had the slightest interest in becoming. I volunteered with Cambodian refugees in the United States and on the Cambodian border. No matter what was going on in their lives, they went to the doctor and would bring everything there, but the doctor would also have something to give. I ended up thinking, Is this the right profession? I could be an anthropologist, but would that truly help them? I went off to medical school, I did residency and fellowship. It was this tremendous process that took time and energy. By the time I finished, I felt like, yes, I had these skills to give to people. And I was interested in people. But parts of me had been lost. I did a few different things, I took a lovely vacation and adopted a dog. I took two classes at the UC Extension in graphic design and mystery novel writing. I think we all need something that nourishes us and connects us to who we were before we were doctors. It is who you can still be, but not if you don't pay attention to it. I always wanted to do X. At this point, I was a dud. Finally, I realized, either you have to do what you love, or you need to stop talking about it. I started writing, really thinking it would be my extracurricular activity. Actually, there was no pressure because I was pretty bad at it. One of the other terrific advantages of medicine is you know you are doing important work, you make a good salary, you get health insurance, you get social respect and acknowledgment. Those things might have helped me be a writer initially. I could let myself enjoy this thing that I really enjoyed, like anyone else's extracurriculars. I just loved the learning of it and

the creativity. I initially thought that I would write this structured, lengthy novel. But my life was so much about stories. I had heard so many stories, and I wasn't getting to tell or process or see the stories. Thus they just naturally became something important I needed to work through and on.

I was writing about doctors and patients and I started to bring it in to my career. They could have stayed separate; they fulfill different essential enterprises and roles in society. Yet I was so involved with nurses, patients, their families, that my gregarious outward-facing self led me to want to engage with their lives more, in a creative way, in what I hoped for them. Then it surprised me; it became even more exciting when all the parts came together, when I began compulsively writing. Then I met medical students and residents who didn't want to write but had something to say. Are we all going to be Atul Gawande? Maybe not. But doctors are smart people and when we have something to say, it needs to get out there and have an impact. I wanted to make that impact and help others do it too, and thus writing became a part of my medical career. Long story short, I was this compulsive doctor who needed to write, so I developed a field called narrative advocacy to improve health and medical care, and to engage with others. You can use narrative advocacy is so many different ways: you can advocate for research work on a particular disease, or you can better process a case clinically. There are great, amazing things you can do with stories and writing. The biggest pleasure in my life is that I get to meet people and hear and tell their stories. The most inspiring part of earning a medical degree is that you have the chance to do this every day for the rest of your life. Life is incredible. Don't forget that.

a lens into your life - So today I had a 102 year old with a cigarette in her mouth as I, her geriatrician, stood right in front of her face. She has no desire to stop smoking, and I don't want to stop her. Just live. At 102, she should do what she wants.

On a recent great day, I started by working on an article, kind of an advocacy article related to geriatrics, that I encountered as a patient myself. I made huge progress on my article, which is always a good start. I wrote about how medical students need to learn to take care of older people. We all learn to take care of kids, we all learn to take care of babies, but your average medical student will never learn to take care of older people. If you are reading this, please make an effort to learn in medical school. Then I taught critical reflection to our first year medical students here at UCSF, the skill of working through when something is unclear and how to come up with a plan to do better next time by reflecting and analyzing. I also gave a talk to the first years. I love teaching. When a teaching session goes well, that's just really fun. It is nice when they are interactive too, new first year students' enthusiasm for their careers is so great. And teaching them good reflective writing skills is not just an extra thing. It correlates to not getting in trouble in medical

school and scoring highly on boards. Then I had a great team meeting and tried to help our health system here at UCSF take better care of older patients by making our team more interactive and developing new ways of communication. It's really fun. I'm all about being creative and transforming. Subsequently, I met with a junior faculty member who is going to have a new leadership position and also a couple of articles. The biggest issue for her was: Now that I am a success, how do I manage these things with two small children? As her mentor, I hope to help her find that balance.

The most exciting part of this day was leading my new initiative to help doctors give bad news and have appropriate conversations with their patients in the face of great suffering. I believe it is a skill that can be taught, just as tools are taught in surgery. Teaching doctors to think about their inner feelings and reflect on their professional behavior can make our role in people's lives more righteous and ethical. And I've learned that if you can change a certain number of people, then the transformed structure will change the rest.

At the end of the day, I ask myself, did I turn off everything else in the presence of my patients? Did I turn off everything and focus just on them? I think you have to turn off everything to get something. Part of that is about paying attention, that good feeling. Did something that matters to them that matters in my life too come forward? That helps me better care for them through some shared humanity. If you can truly understand, if you can truly understand, you can truly find meaning. So many people need you, and you can truly change their lives.

Martin Finkel

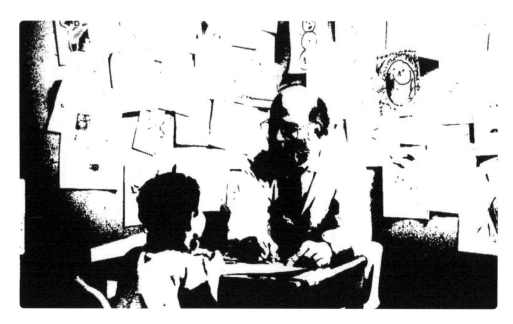

Martin Finkel, D.O. is Professor of Pediatrics at the Child Abuse Research Education and Service (CARES) Institute at the University of Medicine and Dentistry of New Jersey, School of Osteopathic Medicine.

our white coat – A white coat represents a tabula rasa for giving permission for patient to tell and for doctors to listen. It represents permission for doctors to listen and try to understand, so patients can heal. It represents an opportunity for a patient to tell their wholly personal story. The doctor's responsibility is to learn that story.

attending to the world - As a child abuse pediatrician I attend to understand a child's experience filtered by their fears and uncertainty. I am fortunate to attend to children throughout the world by helping doctors understand child sexual victimization and how to respond through publications and lectures. I understand sexual abuse because children shared their frequently shameful, stigmatizing and embarrassing experiences. I listened with empathy and a non judgmental demeanor.

a loving smile - Patience, understanding and compassion provide permission to release emotions, provide relief and generate a smile. Trusting bonds develop as a result of the manner in which the doctor engages with the patient.

a life apart - When I listen I absorb the heartache, when I respond I relieve the heartache. It is the relief I can provide that diminishes my heartache and allows me to continue. I am energized by every child that I see. They validate the value I can bring to their care, I am not sad.

a story - Healing only begins when children share their innermost secrets and fears. My barometer for healing is when a child no longer fears to share and their confused/distorted perceptions of an experience are corrected.

a lens - This image is from the early days of my work and captures the essence of how I learned to help children suspected of experiencing sexual abuse: engaged listening.

additional thoughts on my career -
I am a professor of pediatrics who stumbled on the issue of child sexual abuse 31 years ago when this issue was just appearing on societies radar screen. I have dedicated my professional career to understanding the medical diagnosis of child sexual abuse and building systems of intervention and protection. I am an internationally recognized authority and have contributed much to the understanding of the medical diagnosis of child sexual abuse. I have been honored to be able to do this work on behalf of children.

Mayer Davidson

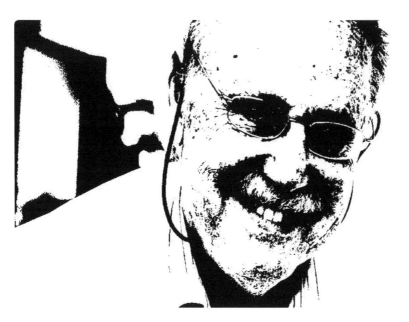

Mayer B. Davidson M.D. is Co-Founder of the non-profit organization Venice Family Clinic. He is a Professor of Medicine at the Charles R. Drew University School of Medicine with an in-residence appointment at the David Geffen School of Medicine at University of California, Los Angeles. He is the Director of the Diabetes Program in the Martin Luther King-Multiservice Ambulatory Care Center (MLK-MACC).

our white coat – In my specialty, diabetes, patients are really the healers. All we can do is to educate, motivate, and suggest (i.e., prescribe) what they should do to heal, or in the case of diabetes, prevent the potential devastating complications of the disease. There is an old saying: You can lead a horse to water, but you cannot make him drink. In that scenario, if patients drink, they "heal" themselves.

attending to the world – In counseling and treating patients, it is most helpful to see the world through their eyes. Rather than setting ourselves apart (read "over them") and simply telling patients what they should do, the physician is much more effective seeing the problems through their eyes and trying to address their issues (to the extent possible) as one treats them.

a loving smile – Practicing medicine is often repetitious and not very intellectually stimulating. The satisfaction comes from becoming involved with patients and their families, i.e., bonding with them. They need to know that you really care about them over and beyond their particular medical problems.

a life apart – When one of your patients dies, of course one feels sad. But let's be frank, we start building our protective (intellectual) walls in medical school so that we can move on and continue to take care of our patients after we lose one. Frankly, it can be a little isolating, but it's totally necessary. The challenge is not to have that wall spill over into our personal lives.

Michael Gisondi

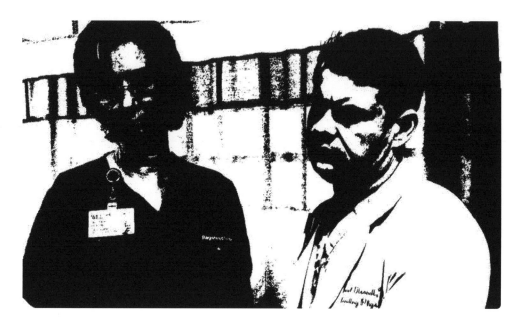

Michael A. Gisondi M.D. is Associate Professor of Emergency Medicine and Emergency Medicine Residency Program Director at The Feinberg School of Medicine at Northwestern.

our white coat - The white coat was a source of great stress for me when I was in medical school. I never liked wearing it. During my pre-clinical years, we had occasional opportunities to shadow physicians on the wards or in clinic. I would look forward to those afternoons, until the moment arrived when I donned my white coat. I felt uncomfortable as soon as I put it on.

I likened the weekly ritual to Halloween, as I felt that I was in costume. I knew very little about medicine then. I certainly had not yet earned the confidence patients seemed to have in me, simply because I was wearing a lab coat. What accomplishments deserved their trust? Taking tests and gaining entrance into medical school? That wasn't enough for me to feel that I belonged at their bedside. And the white coat made it worse. Upon entering clerkships, the coat was figuratively and literally heavy – I was that student who carried a half-dozen study guides crammed into my pockets… before the days of smart phones. Invariably those review books would fall out of my pockets at the most inopportune times, reminding me and everyone around me that I was dependent on my peripheral brains. I still wasn't experienced enough to deserve the coat. Just when I thought I mastered the delicate balance of full pockets that didn't empty onto the ground, I became an intern and my coat got longer. However, with a longer coat came the title of "Doctor" and a steep learning curve that brought me much-needed confidence. By second year of residency I had shed the coat, shirt and tie – in favor of scrubs, my preferred professional garb. As I reflect on my transitions through medical school and residency, the white coat served as a challenge. A challenge by my patients and society to earn the right to wear it, the right to call myself a physician, and the right to tend to acutely ill and injured patients in the emergency department. Those patients, through blind trust in a coat perhaps, taught me to be a professional. I don't think twice about wearing a lab coat now – mine is grey, in distinction to the white coat of our students and house staff – it is ritual, but no longer costume.

attending to the world - Rightly or not, the emergency department is considered by many to be the safety net of the American healthcare system. It is unclear when that role will change for the specialty of emergency medicine. However much I support healthcare reform, I'm not sure that I want reforms to change my role in the safety net. I take immense pride in knowing that my colleagues and I will care for any patient, of any ethnic or socioeconomic background, for any complaint, at any time of day, regardless of their ability to pay for treatment. That is the definition of public service that I was raised to understand by my parents, a mother who was and ER nurse and a father who was a firefighter. Many a holiday did I only have one parent at home, while the other was on duty at work. Many an evening dinner, the same situation. As I matured, I recognized what their absence embodied: my family's commitment to others. I can't pretend that I entered medicine with such admirable intentions – I don't think that my parents had charitable ambitions when they took their jobs either. But it takes a certain personality to be an ER doc, a nurse, a fireman, a police officer, a teacher… we come from a similar mold, we provide care and advocacy for others, and we come to love our respective callings. I do.

uplifting the medically underserved - Healthcare is a human right due to one by society. It may not always have been so, but in an era of technology and collective wealth our responsibility to one another has fundamentally changed. A counter-response, to leave someone who is ill in need, is simply inhumane. It may be irresponsible of me to not more loudly message that belief. I'm convinced that healthcare reform will come only through the shouting of the medical profession to demand policy change. I occasionally wonder if I have a societal responsibility to publically advocate for such change... to shout. Perhaps I fall short because I don't seek to personally enact political change. Instead, I view my skills and abilities to be best used in direct patient care and the instruction of future physicians. I'm a cog in the wheel of the system. I hope an important cog though, especially for the patients who seek my care in times of great need. Medical professionals choose to lead in a variety of ways. America needs physician leaders engaged in political debate to advance policy and healthcare reform. She also needs physicians assigned to the bedside of our people, to ensure that care is accessible and equitable to the extent that it can be in our current system. This is my role, my contribution to the process.

a loving smile - My ability to strike a connection with my patients has changed over my career. When I finished residency, patients and their family members routinely commented on how young I appeared. I knew that such statements were never a compliment, rather they represented a polite acknowledgement that the patient had doubts about my abilities and I needed to work for their trust. I learned very quickly that certain communication techniques were critical to establishing a relationship with my patients; sitting down, taking time to listen, respectfully acknowledging pain and suffering, smiling, holding hands. These were my tools. The older I appear, the less effort I spend establishing such trust - but ever more effective are these communication techniques. They allow me to quickly bond at a much different level. I

share my own life experiences more frequently now, such as the death of my mother and the birth of my daughter, to provide a connection and to contextualize my sympathy and empathy. I call patients at home to check on them too; I never did that when I was first in practice. I worry about my patients in different ways now -- much less concern for misdiagnoses, much more preoccupation with their overall well-being. Age and experience have strengthened my relationships with patients, setting new expectations for myself and those that I serve.

a life apart - Feel sad. Feel sad when situations deserve your sorrow. You are human, first. In medicine, sorrowful situations can become routine. Routine allows us to cope. Scripting and practice allow physicians to routinely break bad news or provide death notifications to survivors. Intellectual engagements with our colleagues allow us to routinely redefine the bizarre and tragic as 'interesting cases.' We are distanced from the rest of humanity by the coping mechanisms we learn during our professional development. Though distanced, we are still human. At the end of every resuscitation, successful or not, I try to thank each member of the emergency department staff who played a role - residents, students, nurses, techs, pharmacists, chaplains, paramedics... and when I do so, I look at their faces. I attempt to recognize when my co-workers are unable to emotionally distance themselves from the chaos they attended. When recognized, those staff members need my immediate attention and a team debrief.

However, providers are often skilled at hiding their natural human responses… of hiding grief, sadness. They keep their masks on and continue with their duties. Seemingly strong providers slowly carry much emotional burden. As the team leader, I put my mask on first. Have my co-workers occasionally seen me cry on shift? Yes, when I can no longer carry the burden alone. Do I show those emotions regularly? No, for practical requisites of leadership as much as pride. My secret is to cry in my car on the way home -- an unfortunately common and likely suboptimal method of addressing the emotions of my practice. But when I finish, I am reminded that I am still human.

a story - One of the saddest, yet inspirational and instructive patients I have cared for was the second patient I encountered on my first medical school clerkship. I use the phrase, "cared for" loosely – as I recall, all that I did was write a note in the chart. Otherwise I was an observer of care provided by others, a student bearing witness to true human tragedy. 'General surgery' was my first clinical rotation, though my initial two weeks were assigned in the Burn ICU. On the first day with that service, a thirty-something year-old male employee of a local steel mill was brought by helicopter to our burn center after a chemical explosion. His burns were so extensive that he most certainly would die that day. Facial swelling made for a difficult intubation en route to our hospital, so he was still conscious and in obvious agony. I watched as my attending compassionately provided his prognosis to the patient within minutes of his arrival. Their joint decision was to forgo intubation so that the patient could remain awake in order to say good-bye to his wife and children, who were less than an hour away from our facility. I watched. I watched as his respiratory distress worsened, his pain seemed uncontrollable. I watched as tears fell into his facial wounds while telling his wife that he loved her. I watched as my attending then sedated the patient and fiberoptically intubated him with family at his bedside. I watched as he died that evening. Later, I found the call room for the first time and I closed the door and I cried. Why is such an awful story both inspirational and instructive? For me, I learned much about the human spirit that day. Healers can do profound work, even if their healing actions can't stave off death. I practice a medical specialty in which I sometimes save lives. However over the years, I have tried to become skilled at recognizing when life can't be saved, but death can be made less awful for patients and their families. Rarely do I see terminally-ill patients who have made peace with their condition. Generally, death is awful. I witnessed an awful death that day in the burn unit. But there was poetic beauty in the love of a dying husband saying an unexpected farewell to his young wife. And there was beauty in the way he was cared for by my attending. I will never forget that patient.

a lens into your life - Emergency medicine is not always exciting – and rarely does my practice resemble what is glamorized on television.

Not to be mistaken, I think adrenaline-filled shifts are wonderful. Most emergency physicians find great professional satisfaction when they encounter complex, challenging cases that draw on their resuscitative skills and training. Those make for great days. Emergency physicians are gifted story tellers, mostly because we have seemingly unlimited stories. I recount my unusual cases to others with great enthusiasm. Though when I get home and start describing my day, my daughter is generally not impressed with the gore of one story or my intellectual abilities on display in another. She is six years-old and she is very wise. She usually cuts me off and simply asks, "Daddy, did you fix someone today?" My best days are when I can truthfully respond, "Yes."

Pablo Hernandez-Itriago

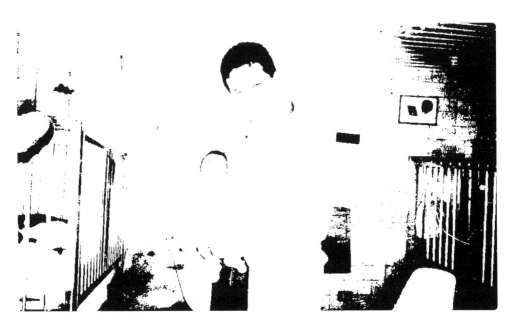

Pablo Hernandez-Itriago, M.D. is Clinical Associate Professor in the Department of Family Medicine at the Boston University School of Medicine and Medical Director at the South End Community Health Center.

our white coat - The white coat can be a powerful barrier, but if you don't interrupt and let the patient finish his first sentence, he will give you the diagnosis.

attending to the world - Once in a while I see a former student or resident, and it is amazing to hear the healing they are doing around the world. It is humbling to get recognition of being part of those formative moments.

a loving smile - Even in the worst of times, we (my patient and I) can find something to laugh about. I have a patient who always tells me, what he loves the most is that no matter how much pain he has, when he comes to the office he knows the laughter will make him feel better.

a life apart - I was born in Venezuela. It was hard when I realized I was not going back anytime soon. Once you make a decision, you need to keep going, seek what is on the other side of the tunnel, have fun. Your best moments are yet to come, starting with today!

a story - He was just a couple of years older than me. He and I knew he was going to die from cancer. Our job was to help his family go through the difficult journey to a premature end. I saw her months after he died. She just said thank you. I knew then, we had done a good job.

a lens - This photo was given to me by the mother of the child I am holding. I was on my last year of medical school. The baby girl almost died from dehydration, we saved her.

I was set to become a surgeon. At the end of medical school, I knew I wanted to be a family doctor, but life had it that I would start my residency in Surgery. After two years, I was able to switch to Family Medicine. Since finishing my residency, working at a community health center, it's just natural to me - I don't see it any other way. We provide high quality care to all who need it. When I cannot find the cure, I always remember the aphorism "To cure sometimes, to relieve often, to comfort always."

Patch Adams

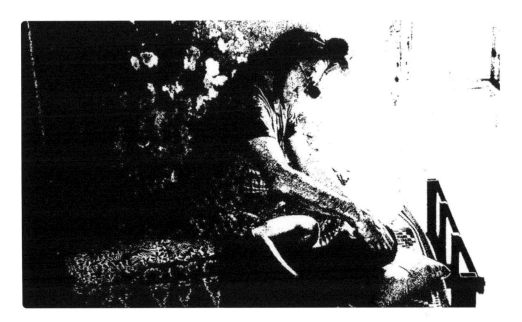

___ is the Founder of the Gesundheit Free Clinic in the West Virginia Mountains and the physician upon which the Academy Award-acclaimed film *Patch Adams* is based.

our white coat - I quickly turned in my white coat for my everyday colorful clothes, with toys. I've always been free and gave initial interviews of four hours to bond in friendship with patients.

attending to the world - The health of the world is abysmal and it is essential for the physician to take a lead in peace, justice, and care for all people and nature, or our survival is unlikely. Doctors must be activists.

a loving smile - My ideal patient is someone who wants a deep personal friendship with me for life. In the hospital we are building, we require the staff to be happy, funny, loving, cooperative, creative, and thoughtful.

a life apart - I chose as a political art to be happy all the time. I think the emotions are all good - the sense organs of the mind - so I do feel sad over the capitalist system, violence, and injustice, and my mind positions me as a radical activist.

a story - I just got back from an annual two week Russian clown trip - and on a burn ward - spent one and a half hours with a five year old [who had been] in the hospital for one year. He had not done any speaking after the fire. After intense fun, play, and toys, he spoke twice.

Rachel Remen

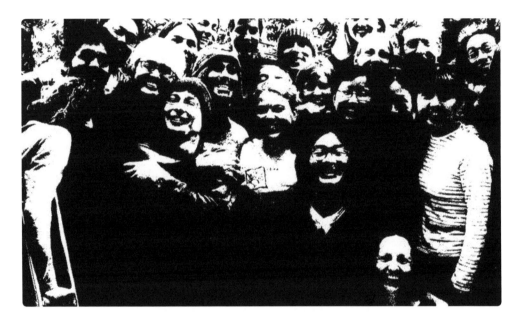

is a pediatrician and medical educator and one of the pioneers of Integrative Medicine and Relationship Centered Care. She is a Clinical Professor of Family and Community Medicine at the University of California, San Francisco School of Medicine. Her discovery model course for medical students on the art of medicine, The Healer's Art , is now taught annually in more than half of America's medical schools as well as medical schools in Taiwan, Israel, Slovenia, Australia, India, Brazil, and Canada. Dr. Remen is a master storyteller and author. *Kitchen Table Wisdom* and *My Grandfathers Blessings*, her *The New York Times* best-selling books on medicine, service, and healing, have been translated into 21 languages.

our white coat - Actually, we are all healers. Curing is the work of experts, but healing is the work of human beings. Long before there were experts people were healing one another, strengthening the will to live in one another with their listening, their belief, their caring, and their willingness to accompany others into dark places. Cure is about the recovery of physical function. Healing is about the recovery of a life, the recovery of a dream of yourself, the strength and courage to live beyond physical limitations and contribute and love. When we heal someone we move them closer to an unsuspected wholeness and possibility in them, a greater sense of identity and personal value. We enable them to live larger and be larger than they were before they met us. Human beings have been doing this for one another for thousands of years. We all wear white coats.

attending to the world - Service is not a technique or a skill or a competency. Service is a way of life. Service is a relationship between equals. When we "help" we may see others as weaker, when we "fix" we may see others as broken, but when we serve we see others as equals, as fellow human beings. We help with our strength, we fix with our expertise, but we serve with ourselves, our wholeness, our common humanity. In 50 years of doctoring I have found that everything I know and everything I am can serve to evoke the wholeness in others, to remind them of their own possibility. We do not need to be perfect in order to serve others: our own pain and limitation have taught us compassion for the pain and limitation of others. Our woundedness and losses make us gentle with the wounds of others and and able to trust the mysterious process by which wounds and losses heal, not as a theory but through our own lived experience. Our loneliness helps us to recognize the loneliness in others despite the masks that people wear, to find others who

have become frightened and alone in the dark and be there with them. Our human vulnerability means that no one who is vulnerable need feel small or ashamed in our presence. We are enough just as we are to heal others.

bonding with patients - We bond with patients and all other people through a certain kind of listening that is the foundation of the healing relationship. My students call this "Generous Listening." Usually when people listen they are actually very busy and concerned with many questions. Do I like what I am hearing? Do I believe it? Do I like the person who is speaking to me? Is this person like me or not like me? We often listen competitively: is this person smarter than I am or not as smart as I am? More articulate or less articulate? More gifted or lucky or less gifted or lucky? And of course as physicians we are trained to ask ourselves, What is wrong with this person? And do I know how to fix it? And all the while someone is telling us something that means a great deal to them. In Generous Listening we stop doing all these things. We are not even listening in order to understand why another person may feel as they do. We listen simply to *know what matters*, what is important to the person who is speaking. Just to know and accept what is true for them. When you listen to another person in this way they feel seen, accepted, and valuable. They recognize that they are not alone and that you can be trusted with anything they may need to tell you.

a story - In the Healer's Art course, first year medical students have a chance to write a personal Hippocratic oath, a personal statement of their own dream of themselves as a physician and what they hope to offer their patients. One year at UCSF a young man who was a football star in college stood and read the following statement of commitment to his future patients:

May you find in me the Mother of the World.

May my hands be a mother's hands.
My heart be a mother's heart.
May my response to your suffering
be a mother's response to your suffering.
May I sit with you in the dark
as a mother sits in the dark.
May you know through our relationship
that there is something in this world that can be trusted.

For me this statement says it all. After 50 years of doctoring and more than 60 years as a patient with a chronic disease, it has become clear to me that Medicine is not a work of science. Science is only our most recent set of tools. Medicine is a work of Service and service is an act of love.

Rushika Fernandopulle

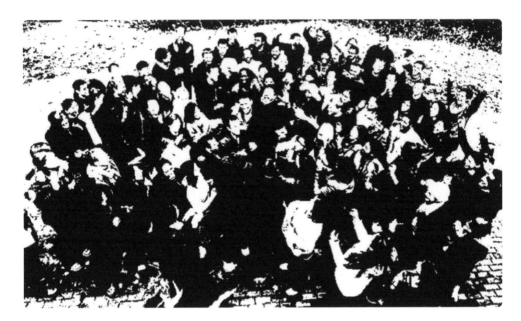

Rushika Fernandopulle M.D. is Co-Founder and CEO of Iora Health, an innovative health care services company based in Cambridge, MA, building a new model of primary care practices nationally. He is Inaugural Executive Director of the Harvard Interfaculty Program in Health Systems.

our white coat - What is interesting to me is that at Iora, we do not wear white coats by design. While I serve on the faculty at Harvard Medical School, and the white coat ceremony is symbolic, unfortunately in real practice it can be-come a barrier that sets the doctor apart with an authoritative, elevated status. This leads me to believe that white coats on the whole can be negative. Because of this, at Iora Health, we do not wear white coats by design. We have a strong belief that the whole notion that I, the doctor, will manage the health of our patients is one in which we are truly fooling ourselves. Two or three hours a year, the patient is in front of us. 8756 hours per year, he or she is not in front of us. The reality is that patients and their family manage health, our job is to provide them with help and resources they need ot do this. I firmly believe that the doctor needs to be a partner and not an authoritative figure. We are just a team of helpers, and the patient is on that team. By engaging with each patient, we improve their health on an individual basis.

One of the things that people notice that is unique about our practice, is that we begin with a huddle. The whole team sits around a table for forty-five minutes. One of the first things people notice, is that people can't tell who the doctor is. The doctor does not run the huddle, everyone takes turns running the huddle, including not only each nurse but also each secretary.

attending to the world - I think it is our job. I think when we all became doctors, almost everyone took an oath to take care of our patients. I think that you learn pretty quickly that if all you do is take care of one patient at a time, you will not be able to do that, because the system is so screwed up. If you don't make an impact on the system, you can't succeed. It isn't an either or; it is about both ends. Take care of individual patients and use that to change the world. You can do that in a variety of ways. I have chosen to rebuild the system of primary care. We have a unique chance as a physician to bear witness to what is happening in our patients' lives—to try to fix the world as well as take care of people.

uplifting the medically underserved - Healthcare is a basic human need, similar to food and shelter, etc. It is in that group of things. The way I think we need to frame it is as a collective responsibility. I think that this phrase in the con-text of natural rights is not useful. The natural rights to free speech, that someone should not infringe upon my free speech, and should not infringe upon my religion, these make sure that the public doesn't do something. A right to healthcare is complicated because it means that someone actually has to do something. A more useful framing is that it is a collective responsibility—like for food, education, shelter, and healthcare. I think we have to figure out what that really means and make it happen. Several years ago I had the fortune to lead a project on how to focus the public on the uninsured in America. One of the best ways I felt to help people without health insurance is to tell their stories. Often the most marginalized don't have a voice. We need to all be medical anthropologists, setting their stories back in line with policy. Many of the people are poor and underserved. We need to give them what we believe good healthcare ought to be. It is an ethical obligation. Our current models for caring for the poor don't work. Despite good intentions, we too often simple ask people to take a number and make them wait a long time, and too often the care lacks dignity, is fragmented and reactive and leads to suboptimal outcomes. What I have been working on now is how do we build new models of care delivery for the underserved? How do we provide good care with dignity to people of all walks of life at a low price? How do we do it now?

a loving smile - I think it is essential to bond with a patient. Yet, there are obviously limits to that. A professional relationship should not be an inappropriate relationship. I think, going back to the empathy answer, if one is empathetic one is by definition bonding with patients. It is good for patients, and it is also good for you. If you don't want to bond with patients, well you could have been a researcher at a bench. There is such great joy in you, in each student and doctor, and if you are going to call yourself a doctor, all-in-all, you have to share that with people. You have to have meaningful relationships with the patients and families who depend upon you.

a life apart - I actually think that you have to be human. The second you lose that, you compromise values. We, at Iora, think that certain values are really important, our number 1 is empathy. If you could just get empathy right, the rest follows. You're going to get sad; it is absolutely fine to get sad. I believe that the appropriate response to getting sad is to think about what you can do about it. Today, most physicians either defend or they complain. Complaining is not a productive response. We created this stupid system, we can fix it. And if you don't ever show emotion around a trainee, well, without empathy you missed the point of medical education.

a story - What we do for a living, here at Iora, is we build these new models of primary care practice–a different payment model, a different relationship model. We have health coaches, electronics health records that are patient-centered and not just focused around coding and billing like most. What is it that makes the difference? The story I would like to share is having a patient at our clinic in New Jersey who was completely out-of-control. Her hair was messy, blood pressure high, and sugar immensely out of control as well. She was not going to work, just a mess. We joined one of our practices, and six months later she was a new person, hair combed, blood pressure under control, no emergency room visits anymore. I looked her in the eye, and asked, "what have we done to make you feel better?" She said, "You all cared about me, and you taught me to care for myself. I didn't want to let either of us down." We have forgotten that in healthcare, we now have a series of transactions and billing, yet healthcare is all about human interaction. Whether someone cares about you and helps you care about yourself. If we can get that right, the rest will definitely follow.

a lens into your life - I don't have an average day. Every day is different, yesterday for instance, I was in Las Vegas, Nevada visiting a practice of ours. I started out having a huddle with our team, talking about patients coming in, who we needed to help and reach out to. I spent a couple hours with them. Then I went to the hospital to visit a couple patients in the hospital, talked about how we could work together better. I had dinner with some of our team, and took the red-eye flight back to Boston. The next morning, after landing, I led the opening of a training session at Harvard Medical School. Ultimately, later in the day I reviewed proficiencies of our clinics, and then headed to our clinic in Dorchester. I like when I get to constantly be involved in making an impact 24/7.

At the end of the day, it's all about treating patients as people, as people like you and me. If you forget who people are, turn in your white coat.

Gurpreet Dhaliwal

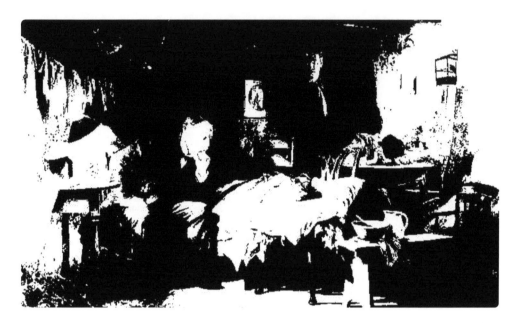

Gurpreet Dhaliwal M.D. is Professor of Medicine at UCSF. He is an expert in clinical reasoning and was featured in *The New York Times* as one of the nation's leading diagnosticians.

our white coat - The white coat serves as an outward manifestation of our profession, but our professionalism is manifested through words and actions. You show that you're a professional by displaying respect, dedication, and compassion.

attending to the world - A physician works in service to his or her patients, trainees, colleagues, and society. Service to society includes being a good steward of finite health care resources and making decisions that take into account the patient in front of me today but also the patient in front of me tomorrow. As doctors, we are indebted to society, family, teachers, and all the patients we learn from. We wouldn't have become doctors without them. This is the greatest job in the world. The ability to do work that's so intellectual, so humanistic, so valued - that's a very unique combination that we're incredibly privileged to be able to do.

uplifting the medically underserved - Health care is a human right. I believe all members of society are entitled to safety, education, and health care. When those three rights are assured, human beings flourish. I work in a health care system that provides full access, the VA system, which is amazing in the breadth of care it provides at no or low cost to our veterans. We still have to navigate the system for our patients, but we do so equitably without regard to race or socioeconomic status. Everyone needs a health coach and should get the care they deserve.

We're in the service of the patient, I really believe that point so strongly. The real mark of a professional is someone who puts the patient's interest before his or her own.

a loving smile - A bond will be formed immediately if you're in the service of a patient. The bond signifies that I'm working on your behalf. I'm invested in a good outcome for you, not necessarily for me. I'm happy to meet you, you may not be happy to meet with me (understandably – who likes to go to the doctor?), but the two of us are going to make the best of the situation. We don't have to be friends, but it should be friendly. A smile is the universal gesture of kindness. If a smile comes naturally when you interact with patients, then you're in the right job.

a life apart - Living as a human being and living as a doctor together inform your sense of empathy. You see the spectrum of the human condition - the amazing triumphs and the heartbreaks. Empathy is recognizing the emotion and experience of another human being. Sadness is more of feeling the emotional pain yourself. I wouldn't say you have to experience sadness in this job, but you must have a sense of empathy. You need empathy to effectively operate on patients' behalf and be able to choose the right course for them. If you can't put yourself in their shoes, then you can't do right by them. If we don't read our patients' emotions, feel their pain, or understand their world, we can't succeed in the fundamental tasks of advising them or making the best decisions for them. Two patients may be identical biologically but be in different emotional states, and that calls for different advice, a different talk, and a different plan for each.

a story - The stories that stick with me are the mistakes I made. Sometimes they're minor, sometimes they're major, and sometimes they've harmed patients. Those are the cases that make me a better physician, so I keep track of those instances. We're in the improvement business. We are wired to improve patients' health outcomes, but we increasingly have to think about improving our own performance and that of the health care system. In some sense it's okay to make mistakes, it's just not okay to not learn from them. In the practice of medicine, there's too much variability in the human condition to eliminate mistakes and bad outcomes, but we should continually endeavor to minimize them. In this profession we have to be okay with uncertainty and helping patients navigate uncertainty. I always examine my performance. Maybe I did the best I could today, but I'll aim to do better tomorrow.

On motivation to become a physician - My parents are physicians. They are extraordinarily happy physicians who have just finished their 40th year of practice as allergists in Kenosha and Racine, Wisconsin. There's no doubt that having parents in medicine had an effect, but it was a background rather than foreground influence on my career choice. I entered a combined seven year undergraduate-medical school program out of high school. However, like all students, I had no idea what being a doctor really entailed until I entered the clerkship years. It's a leap of faith when you sign up.

When I got in, I asked, Can it really be this great? That you get to work in a job that's intellectually challenging, that plays an important role in society, and involves day-to-day contact with amazing people. When you step back it almost boggles the mind that there is a profession where you get to experience that on a daily basis. I suspect I was attracted to the intellectual challenges first, but later the joys of combining teaching and healing really appealed to me, and now it's the relationships that I have with patients and trainees and colleagues that are the most sustaining part of my career.

On learning from patients - Patients have taught me a lot. Sometimes it's frank feedback, things that I didn't want to hear, such as, "You told me something and it didn't wind up being true." But the bigger lessons are the daily demonstrations of the human capability to face adversity. I'm fortunate not to have had a major health event in my life. When that times comes, I'd like to think I will handle it with the grace, fortitude, and optimism that my patients have demonstrated as they faced their tragedies. This profession gives you a window into how amazing humans can be and the capacity of people to respond to life's greatest challenges. I have the extra privilege of taking care of people who have served the United States in the military. At this hospital, it's not only our duty to serve them but an honor to serve them. I regularly treat veterans who have faced amazing challenges in the theatre of war, and in another stage of their life are facing an equally if not more harrowing episode. When you enter the VA hospital you will see this quote: "The price of freedom is visible here." That really inspires me and reminds me that every society needs brave men and women, who now are in our care, in order to enjoy all the privileges and liberties we have in our society.

On mentors - In medical school at Northwestern University, my most cherished mentor was Robert Hirschtick, MD. I now have the same role that he did (and still does) when I was a student: the VA Internal Medicine Clerkship Site Director. He was the embodiment of a master clinician: great intellect, superb bedside skills, and unfailingly with a smile on his face. To my eye he was always in the service of his patients and his trainees. In him I saw a model of what a clinician educator was and knew that that role was something I could aspire to. When I came to UCSF, I worked with Lawrence Tierney, M.D., who remains my mentor to this day. He too personifies the master clinician. In him I see a combination of medical knowledge, bedside manner, and teaching ability that I might never see the likes of again.

On being a master diagnostician - It's a side effect of a career spent studying medicine with an active clinical practice and then studying the diagnostic process. Getting good at diagnosis (I won't accept "master") takes years and years of studying two things: the canon of medical knowledge and how the mind works. Being cognizant of ways to train the brain to excel and cognizant of ways you can avoid pitfalls are two things that can help you recognize common diseases in typical and atypical manifestations, and when lucky, pick up rare diseases that usually evade our attention. You have to study how the body works to be good, and you should study how the mind works to be great. It's metacognition: thinking about thinking. After a case, I perform a cognitive autopsy; I go back and analyze my own thinking to reflect on what I or my team did right, but also where we went wrong.

On being compared to Dr. House - I'm not as smart as him, but I'm much nicer than him.

When we define a master clinician today they should have both intellectual firepower and a heart of gold. You have to have the two together to earn the title "master clinician." Dr. House lacked the latter. If you want to be a master clinician, you have to work at both aspects of physicianship. The two feed off of each other. No one is interested in a doctor who is good at one and neglects the other.

On changes in medicine - I would really like to see everyone in the country and the world have access to health care. The way we do health care has to be improved. We could do health care more effectively, efficiently, and safely. I hope to see it in my lifetime. What I'd really like also is for the medical system to be a health system. Right now it's set up to react to illness. To focus on maintaining and restoring health would be a major advancement. Our tolerance for bad outcomes is still too high. The entire health care system is too complicated - from regulations to paperwork- and there are too many things that stand between the simple goal of a doctor trying to improve the health of the patient.

a lens into your life - *The Doctor* (1891), by Sir Luke Fildes. What I find quite inspiring is the physician solely focused on and dedicated to his patient. He's not doing anything at the moment, but that bespeaks a secret of medicine: just being present and caring is the essential element of being a doctor. That you are there and that you care. The picture captures it in a way that few writings and images can. *(Editor's Note: This image is featured on Dr. Dhaliwal's cover page).*

Resident and Student Leaders

Daniel Nagasawa

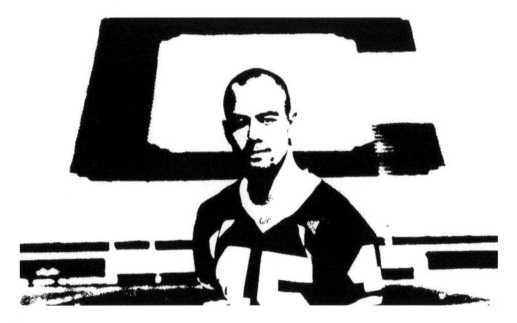

Daniel Nagasawa, M.D. is a Neurosurgery Resident at University of California, Los Angeles Medical Center and former wide receiver for the University of California, Berkeley football team.

our white coat – When I was given my short white coat as a medical student, I was so excited to put it on; it was my initial step into medicine, symbolic of taking on the role of being a student physician for which I had worked so hard to become. The transition to wearing the long white coat was even more powerful, repre-

senting my transformation into an individual responsible for patient education and improvement of health. When patients see that coat, they see someone they are willing to trust with their lives.

attending to the world - From the moment we first put on that white coat in medical school, our lives became devoted towards improving the wellbeing of others, regardless of socioeconomic class, gender, religion, or any other status. Whether it is through direct medical care, patient education, or public policy, we are here to help anyone who walks through the hospital doors.

a loving smile - I think a good personality and a loving smile can go a long way. In their greatest times of need, patients will open up to you and tell you some of their deepest secrets and greatest fears. They divulge information openly and honestly in hopes that you will express compassion, empathy, and be able to help them through this difficult situation. The things we tell our patients – cutting out organs, drilling holes in their skull, etc- are terribly frightening. Patients need to know that they can trust you, and that you will always have their best interest at heart. That is how you will be able to make a difference in their lives and not just be the one to dictate a best course of action.

a story - The first time I was able to drill a hole for a patient with a subdural hematoma was an incredible experience. The surgery was successful and afterwards, the Attending took me outside the OR, shook my hand, and said, "Welcome to the club." That was a huge moment for me; he was a very prestigious physician who had welcomed me into the world of neurosurgery and accepted me as one of their own.

a lens - I 100% believe that as individuals, experiences throughout our lives (positive or negative) are things we can use to help others. One of my main influences was as a student-athlete at Cal. Playing football and still achieving academic success required a heightened level of commitment, devotion, and discipline. I know I strive to maintain that same level of passion in order to ensure my patients receive the best care our hospital can deliver.

Elana Miller

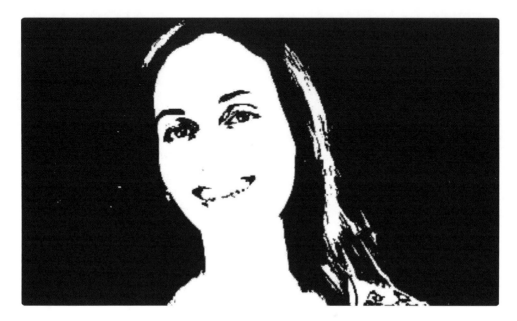

Elana Miller M.D. is Psychiatry Resident at University of California, Los Angeles Medical Center. Elana is currently overcoming, beating, and-destroying stage IV cancer.

our white coat - One of my attending's once said, "Don't work harder than the patient." Because often, you get people that come to you and say, "I'm not going to do anything, I'm not going to change my life at all, just fix me." Of course, that is not going to really work—it's a partnership. The doctor is the expert on medicine but the patient is the expert on their own internal experience. For example in psychotherapy, you are not going to go anywhere if the patient is keeping things from you, or putting on an act. It is up to them to be vulnerable and feel comfortable to do that with that particular therapist and do whatever it takes to get better. There is a lot variability in how much initiative patients take. I believe very strongly in personal responsibility in medicine, I feel as if sometimes patients don't have that. Unfortunately, that is probably related to the paternalistic way that medicine has been. With all of these lifestyle disorders such as diabetes and heart disease, you can't just keep smoking and drinking too much, expect your doctor to change your insulin and then have everything be okay.

I struggled with situations where the psychiatrist has to take away the patient's autonomy because there is a fine line that sometimes we cross in the wrong way. There are so many patients I have treated in the hospital here who are manic or psychotic and you have to hold them and medicate them against their will, and after a week they are better and they are appreciate of what you did. But then there are other people where we did the same thing: we held them involuntarily, we force-medicated them, and I don't think we are doing them a service. There are people who simply have paranoid ways of thinking about the world but do not really have a treatable condition such as schizophrenia where we know medications will help. That's hard because I can imagine how frustrating it would be for a patient, and I think when people make mistakes, it probably contributes to the negative perception of psychiatry. It's really tough, because those rules are needed because people can destroy themselves in ways they would regret if they were in their normal state of mind.

There is unfortunately a negative perception of psychiatry, and I think there are a couple different categories of people who contribute to that. I think Scientologists and its suborganizations are a part of that. They actually protest the APA conference every year, write reviews of psychiatry online, and the most famous example being Tom Cruise telling a post-partum depression patient not to take medications that would help her. Then there are people who have had a personally bad experience with psychiatry–they felt more medicated then they should have been. I do think it is not uncommon for psychiatrists to prescribe medications; although I don't know any psychiatrists who prefer doing that, it is something that comes up because that is the only thing insurance companies will reimburse, which is really unfortunate. One of the things I am really passionate about is to put some common sense in the discussion, because there are such extreme opinions. There is this middle ground, and I think if patients understood where psychiatrists are coming from a little bit more, and the limitations that are on them because of insurance companies, they wouldn't be so frustrated. I care very much about having a positive voice in psychiatry.

a life apart - Whenever you feel sad. I understand there is a need to be professional, and especially, you don't want to be totally losing it and breaking down in front of a patient because that's not going to be useful for them. Likewise, you need to be the leader of the medical students and residents on the team, but how often have you been inspired by someone who was stiff, who was not emotive, who just kind of followed the rules? You're inspired when you see some heart in a person. It could be in the smallest way, like the way they touch the patient, that indicates their caring, and I think it doesn't do patients or doctors a service to put those emotions to the side, because that's what it means to be a human being. This is especially relevant in psychiatry, because I have patients where the most important thing I do for them is listen to them and show that I care. For those patients, I don't have any magical words that I give them that gives them this amazing insight, I just care. Patients are not stupid; they can pick up on what you feel.

For example, in terms of where psychiatry is right now, I always say it is one hundred years behind the rest of medicine. That's because we deal with a very complicated organ–the mind. Of course the field is very preoccupied with gaining a better scientific understanding of mental illness and why medications work. However, psychiatry has this appreciation for heart, for the human spirit, for compassion and what it can do and I just hope we don't forget that as we become more like other fields. I feel that there are similar problems in medicine in general; if you ever read articles in the New York Times about any medically related topic, and you read the comments, people comment that physicians just want to get money, but actually that's not really how it works, especially since most doctors are on salary. There are a lot of misunderstandings about what the daily life of a doctor is like, what the limitations on their practice are like.

It is really expensive for people to be put in this position where they can't get routine care. Patients show up to the ER with end-stage asthma, something that is totally treatable; or breast cancers growing out of the skin, and you are just blown away that that even exists in our country. I think there needs to be a single payer system. As annoying as Medicare is, they do some things right, and it is not right that there are insurance companies making money on providing the least amount of care possible while collecting the most premiums. To me that seems like an incentive structure that is totally wrong. I don't think there should be for-profit insurance companies.

I want to provide education so that, patients too have the knowledge to advocate this stuff. The more information people have the better. There is no appreciation for what things cost, and I think patients need to have an appreciation too for having generic drugs and not demanding the most expensive treatment all the time. I think co-pays should be relevant to the cost of the treatment, and be affordable but sting a little so the patient is reminded of what this costs and not take their healthcare for granted. There are so many people in the geriatric psych unit who have low quality of life. In one particular situation, a patient had really bad dementia but no family members to take care of her, and a conservator comes in and determines what medications she takes and when to go to the hospital. The medical team thought that the patient needed to be made Do-Not-Resuscitate (DNR), but the conservator office had a policy where it could not do that unless the patient went through a number of ethics consults. We were put in a situation where we almost had to put a feeding tube in. A lot of the red tape can be avoided if patients have these end-of-life care discussions earlier, and have power of attorneys.

Attending physicians should share their emotional response with trainees. Of course there is probably a balance in the sense that you don't want your attending breaking down in front of the patient, and you probably don't want them to break down in front of you because they have to be a leader. But when something bad happens, a patient dies or there is a really tragic diagnosis, it doesn't help to not talk about it, so I think an attending who in a gentle way expresses their feelings sets a good example for the emotional intelligence of their trainees. Unfortunately I don't think I can actually remember an attending doing that.

Photograph by Michael Bartosek

Renée Betancourt

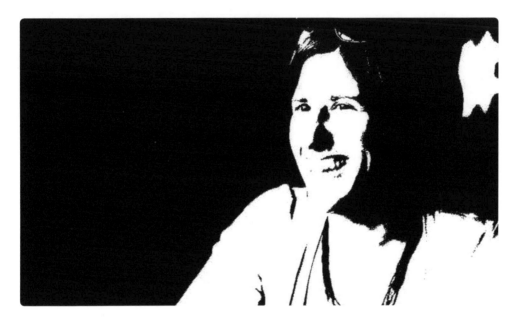

Renée Betancourt M.D. is Chief Resident in the UCSF Family Medicine Residency Program. Dr. Betancourt has included a photo of where she finds beauty and meaning in her life.

our white coat - This white coat is so special to me. As a young woman of color in medicine, my white coat symbolizes that I belong among other physicians and that I have the capacity to provide excellent care for my patients. In academia as well as international and underserved settings, my mentors and my patients may not always be used to seeing women in this role.

The white coat is an instantly recognized symbol of my capacity as a clinician and as an advocate. In the best circumstances, a patient and physician choose one another, based on interpersonal chemistry and the desire to devote time and attention to the well-being of the patient. The physician's white coat is an outward symbol of that intention. My white coat has witnessed a lot of studying, long nights in hospitals away from my family, and some adrenaline-filled moments; and sometimes as a result of all that, it's easy to assume and abuse the inherent power of the white coat. This false sense of control can lead to exhaustion and resentment: "Why won't my patient take his blood pressure medicine? I told him how important it is to prevent another stroke!" I have learned this the hard way. When I remind myself that the patient's decisions are at the center of this work, the act of medicine is joyful and light.

attending to the world - The constellation of privilege and opportunity that has allowed me to become a physician is a joyful debt that I plan to repay through service. For me, practicing medicine among the underserved is a form of practicing justice. I am humbled beyond words to hear about my patients' lives, and I serve as a witness to their obstacles and their triumphs. My goal is to collaborate with my patient in creating a space that holds her story. She gives me the gift of her trust, and I, in turn, hold the burden of her experience for a short while before giving it back to her at the end of a visit. My patients and I come from such different backgrounds, and in most cases, this means that they've lived through traumas that I can just barely imagine after hearing their stories. The medicine is always interesting: diabetes, heart disease, liver disease. But it's the relationship and the trust between us that compels me to return to the clinic so that I can hear more of the story.

a loving smile - A smile, a kiss, a handshake, and a hug are sometimes the only language that my patients and I have in common. After the hours that they often wait for me in a busy clinic, I want them to feel warmth, positive regard, and my attention to whatever they bring to the visit that day. I try to learn the words for "thank you" in all of my patients' languages; if I don't know it, I ask them to teach it to me. At the end of the visit, after I (usually) botch the simple phrase I've attempted to learn, we share laughter as well.

a life apart - I believe that it's important to sit with the sadness that often comes with medicine. Whether it's a young woman who can't kick her addiction and comes in because of an abscess or a cantankerous old veteran receiving a diagnosis of cancer - my own life intersects with some of the more difficult moments in others' lives. I might be dreaming up a grocery list or figuring out what to buy my parents for Christmas when I receive a call from the nurse informing me that our patient has passed away. And so I pivot from the mundane to the most important. In the moment, it feels easy and takes no effort. But sometimes I have trouble making it back to the mundane: I realize I've been staring at the same chips in the grocery store for minutes all the while wondering about my hospice patient. These moments are tough, and I admit to struggling with them. Experienced physicians have taught me the importance of breathing. During a cardiac arrest - take a breath. Before calling a family member to disclose a death - take a breath. When my patient tells me she's been raped - take a breath. Before I walk in the door at the end of the day - take a breath. Breathe in, breath out, and in this

way time goes on. Some sadness I move
through, some I leave behind, and the remain-
der shapes me as a clinician.

a story -
Me: And do you wear your helmet when you
ride your bike?
7 year old girl: <sheepish grin, squirms on ta-
ble> No...
Me: No?! And why not?
7 year old girl: <thinks for a second> Because I
don't have bad luck.
Me: <silence>

Robin Mansour

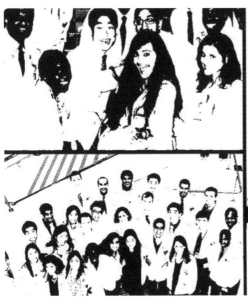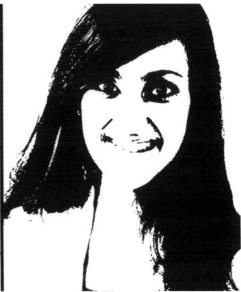

Robin Mansour is Student Body President at the Duke University School of Medicine.

our white coat - Other than avoiding the awkward 'You look young enough to be my granddaughter' comment? Well, from the perspective of the medical student, the white coat gives us the permission and the authority to walk though doors that we would have never normally been able to walk through and to have conversations so private,that we can't even imagine that someone is letting us into their lives and allowing us to see them at their most exposed and vulnerable. The white coat facilitates that. It gives us the ability to be confident in ourselves. When a medical student puts on a white coat, they feel the weight of the profession and the desire to become part of its legacy so that you can become a proficient doctor and be there for people. When medical students start on the wards, they have so little confidence; the first two years don't do an adequate job of preparing you for what it is really like to take care of patients. If you don't have the confidence necessary, then the patients will never open themselves up to you, and you will never do any good for the patient. I think that it may mean something different for a practicing physician, and may be less necessary, because they already have the knowledge, experience, and confidence to do what is needed for the patient.

In a way, the white coat has lost its symbol and meaning for some physicians for pragmatic reasons, like not scaring a child, or otherwise. That hasn't really happened for medical students because for us, it gives us the authority, permission, and confidence we have never had. It represents a burden: the burden of needing to learn impossible amounts of knowledge, of carrying surgical supplies until your neck hurts, and of service. This "burden" is one that medical students wear very proudly, that we get so excited about, and that we attach that to our white coat too.

attending to the world - You walk a fine line between being entirely academic and still meeting the emotional needs of the patient. At the beginning of medical school that might seem forced or contrived. As we progress more, natural displays of empathy become much easier for us. It is just that when you are trying to learn so much and trying to cram, sometimes it takes away from the service that you are doing and from what really matters. Some really active medical students struggle with this concept–investing in ourselves first, and investing in our knowledge, so that one day we can invest in our patients and in our community and give back. Almost like this is our time to focus on ourselves before focusing on the world as a whole.

uplifting the medically underserved - In our day and age, not having access to a physician is a failure of the system at some level and in some way, shape, or form. It is sort of like hunger. It is not that we don't have enough food; food distribution is what needs improvement.

I come from a predominantly immigrant community of Coptic Orthodox Egyptians. We are a Christian community in Egypt, about 10% of the population of Egypt I believe, and are often heavily persecuted, especially during the recent turmoil. Our community has grown over the years, and has become a refugee population. My Dad is a primary care physician in Florida, and he always seems to provide help to those people. People have brought kids to our front door who are feverish. I have seen him always provide service, regardless of capacity to pay or making an appointment or anything like that. I hope to one day be someone who can provide that kind of a link. Also, I hope to do global work in some capacity. Never saying I want to do or I will do. I have never ended up doing what I predicted I would, but I know I want to give back to the community that raised me, and also the global community in some way.

a loving smile - I think an effective physician-leader has a relationship with their patient population on some level. Physicians thatare most real in that one-on-one setting are those who have gotten their patients to make behavioral changes. They are the ones who have a personal relationship with their patients. That personal relationship is what inspires people to really make changes in their lives. So I think I already hammered home the importance of being professional and also personal. If I don't have a personal relationship with my patients, that would take all of the heart out of my job. Otherwise, what's the point really? It's the love for the people I am serving that causes me to serve.

a life apart - I think it is appropriate to feel sad when sad things are happening. I think it's appropriate to feel sad and to acknowledge those sad emotions when something is happening to a patient. Whether you are getting burnt out or whether you have been disillusioned with an ideal, I think it is the people who don't allow themselves to feel sad that just accelerate their burnout. On the flip side, I don't think that sadness should ever be debilitating. I spoke to a resident once who slowly walked out of a room, and sat at her desk. I sat down and asked her questions, and I noticed that she was responding somewhat slowly. I realized that she was trying to hold back tears of emotion rolling up in her eyes. I thought to myself, "I'll let her be," and I walked away. Then she walked away into one of the hospital closets and started crying and she then came out and was able to carry on with the rest of her day. I think needing to take a minute to acknowledge sadness, is a part of being a healthy physician. Because this profession can really, really get to you in your life. Because you are dealing with so many profound

things that have so many implications, you just can't allow them to be paralyzing or crippling.

I like to write about the experiences that I have. I feel like when there is a lot that has happened, I try to hold it all in my mind. If I write it down, I have the opportunity to just say everything that I am thinking. The writing process itself is very cathartic. I talk to a lot of medical students who also share similar experiences. That group process really helps. There is also a course at Duke called Practice Course. We learn about empathy and all the things about being a doctor that doesn't involve medical knowledge. During the second year, it became so much more than showing up for class each week and doing what we usually do. For my group, it became a medical student support group. We laughed and there were times when some of us even cried. It was a really effective coping mechanism, to share and feel unburdened.

I think it is absolutely appropriate for a physician-leader to show emotion in front of their trainees. I think it inspires much more respect, it humanizes them and builds a bond between that trainee and physician, as a mentor, as a colleague; it is those physicians that show the emotion, the one's that show the natural part of being a doctor, the human parts, that end up becoming models and mentors and the one's whom students aspire to be like. It is just so important and cathartic for medical students, who might be feeling a lot of things in the profession for the first time, and who may be confused on how to channel those feelings or what to do with them. It is incredibly healthy for the development of the student. A lot of doctors can look back and tell a story about how a person influenced the entire way that they practice, and it never is usually the physician who is extremely smart and knows everything. It is usually someone that is emotional and deals with the human side of medicine.

a story - I have three favorite stories.

I was on internal medicine and when a medical student starts on internal medicine, it is a huge blow to the face. The variety of information is so overwhelming, no matter how much you study or research or spend time in the hospital, you are confronted with things you have never seen before. Internal medicine is taxing in both an academic and emotional sense. It was the first time that I had to confront end-of-life care issues, telling the family about death, things like that. So I was at the hospital, and there was an older gentleman. He had a mass in his neck, and never went to the doctor for a long time. Finally, he went to the doctor and it was a cancer in his throat; it was inoperable. He was this tiny older man who always winked at everyone when they came into his room, and no matter what, would always crack jokes. His family came to stay with him at the hospital: big, muscular firefighter son and smaller, very compassionate, emotional daughter. And so we would have meetings with the family to discuss end of life care, focusing on quality vs. quantity of years. The question was whether this person

would receive treatment or whether they would decide to just make the patient comfortable and not put him through all of that. The conversations were so long and powerful, and I really learned a lot from them. We all came in the room--attending, residents, medical students--and discussed it for the first time. Listening to this discussion of end-of-life care issues was very difficult for me. I took care of this patient, I checked on him several times per day. The son was a very macho sort of guy, but he just broke down and started to cry. He asked his Dad what he wanted. His dad said, "I have had a great life, gotten to trust and see you kids grow up". I was standing in the back and just started crying silently. I remember sort of being terrified that one of the residents or attendings would pull me out of the room and tell me I should be more professional or stronger. I thought at any moment someone would ask me to leave the room. The PA student sort of squeezed my arm. I remember being quite embarrassed. They ultimately opted for quality over quantity. They discontinued radiation and he went to hospice. As he was leaving, I saw his family one more time. His son gave me this giant hug, and started crying on my shoulder. He thanked me for being the only one to show emotion. He was grateful for something incredibly embarrassing and unprofessional. I was really inspired by that, and learned a lot.

a lens into your life - Ideally, I would be in a community that I know well, because I have invested a lot of time and effort into the community, not just medically but in leadership positions and roles that are important to me outside of medicine. I would like being able to go to the grocery story and church and say hi to people and ask how their children are doing. And I would like to see people in my clinic who have a diversity of backgrounds, languages, and ages. My ideal day would include focus on practice and patients, my community as a whole, and also my family. It would be a balance of all of those things. By being a physician you are usually automatically a leader in your community, but that doesn't just stop with medicine. Ideally I would be involved with my other passions as well. I also would be very involved in the Egyptian community, which is always in need. I think I would probably be one of those people in medicine. I think I would be one of those physicians that would exercise with patients. Oh and like that geriatrician, I'm getting a jet ski in my practice too.

Kristy Hamilton

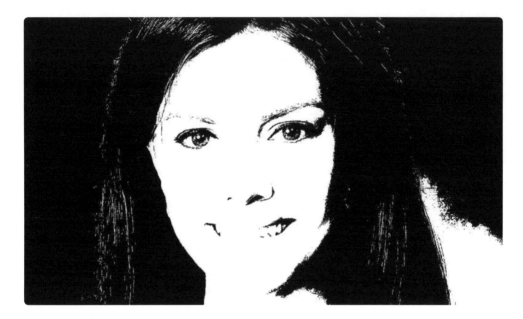

Kristy L. Hamilton is Student Body President at the Baylor College of Medicine. After being interviewed and greatly inspired by the project, Kristy joined the *Service Minded Physician* editorial team.

our white coat - I think that my personal white coat is certainly symbolic. It is a symbol of purity, it is a symbol of the professionalism of what we do. I wear it mainly as a tool. There are some situations where it shows compassion and authority. It comes with heavy responsibility. When I was a first year, during the second week

of medical school we were sent out and knew nothing about medicine. I was twenty-two and I had that white coat on, and everybody referred to me as doctor even though I was introduced as a medical student. I instantly knew I had to be careful about what I said. The patients were going to take whatever I said as informed medical advice. There is this power of the white coat, that makes me treat it with respect. I think there are other times where the white coat can be too intimidating. Pediatric patients are afraid of it, because they associate it with shots. At the same time, it can be the reason some adults talk to us. There are times when I would prefer not to wear my coat and have more of a human-to-human interaction. Yet, I never forget it is a tool and you can use it for healing. Thus there is an important question of when to use and when to leave behind.

attending to the world - Medicine is a service in itself. The idea of a higher calling we all talk about gives me so much purpose. It is so special to get to serve others in this way. It's what gets me up at 4 a.m, excited to go to the hospital, knowing that I can touch and improve people's lives in such an intimate and private way. It is extraordinary and such a privilege that I get to do this. This is the very core of why I am becoming a doctor.

a loving smile - I have a smile on my face everyday, and it is one of the most important tools that I have in my doctor's bag. When you walk into the room with a big smile on your face, when you are enthusiastic when you meet the patients, it sets the patients at ease; it shows them that you care about them. It is an incredible tool for healing and showing that you see them. At the same time it is important to remember that it is not always appropriate. If there is bad news, then it is not the time for something like that. I love smiling; it is a fantastic way to connect with people. Even if people are skeptical a little bit, it forces everyone to let their guard down and at least makes them feel like they can talk to you.

a life apart - I think it is important to always continue to feel those emotions, when you are surrounded by suffering and pain. We are often surrounded by grief and pain, some specialties more than others. Sometimes you have to face the emotions of watching a patient die in front of your eyes or suffer from terminal cancer. Yet, it is okay to know that your patients touch you in this way. It is an important part of continuing to be human. Someone I knew, one of my patients, was going to die. I learned about their life and their family's lives, and I could see everything that they were leaving behind. Everyday it got harder for me and at the end I broke down and cried. With this whole progression you become quite attached. You can't be chirped by it either; you have to find ways where you can continue to take action for the other people who need you, and you have to take care of yourself well. Yet, in this you find meaning, you remember never to refer to patients as "room five" or "the colonoscopy." Patients never become the person getting this or that; they are Mr. and Mrs. Smith. It reminds me of the discussion of physician burnout. I think we prevent it with feelings; feelings give us purpose.

a story - I was 16 and I was shadowing a reconstructive plastic surgeon. I had the chance to observe the operating room, and I was so enthralled with what he could do. Everyone was getting better after each surgery, and then I met one of his patients whom I still remember viv-

idly ten years later. I will never forget this elderly gentleman in a hospital bed. He was eating
his soup and poking at his food. The physician
came in and told him he was going to loose his
foot. I still remember that I was so overwhelmed, I felt like my face was burning. It was
so overwhelming to see this man who was
about to lose his foot. And then the grace with
which he approached it shocked me. He
thanked the doctor. He thanked him for all the
time he spent with him. He was appreciative for
all the care that he had gotten. He smiled and I
could not believe the way he handled that news
and was so strong. It was a big moment in my
life; I was so inspired by his resilience. The way
he handled it without being angry or upset, and
was so kind to everyone else, this is what it
means to be human. I believe that is in everybody.

Amol Agarwal

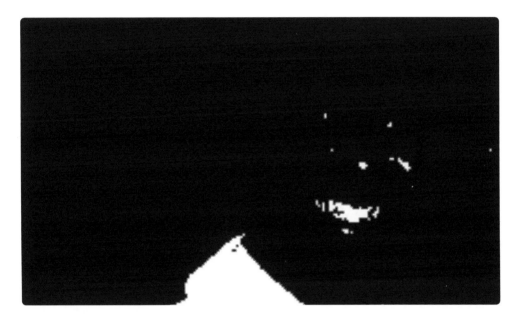

Amol Agarwal is Student Body President at the University of Pennsylvania School of Medicine.

our white coat - In my mind, the white coat is somewhat dichotomous in that it is, on the one hand, a potential barrier to the patient-physician relationship. Patients may see the white coat as representative of them having to give away their privacy and expose their fears to someone else. On the other hand, I also see the white coat as a symbol of what we owe our patients. It endows a sense of humility and really helps remind us what a great role we

have in protecting and promoting the health of our patients. So, while the white coat often symbolizes what is considered the paternalistic nature of medicine of the past, for me it is a welcome reminder of the humbling duty that we have to our patients.

attending to the world - We have a diverse range of healthcare challenges in the 21st century that will have to be tackled in a multitude of ways, from a clinical perspective, from a research perspective, and finally from a policy and advocacy perspective. It cannot be solely up to physicians in positions of power or administrative roles to address these issues; rather, every attending physician, if they are committed to the concept of attending to the world, if they truly are service-minded, must take the burden upon themselves to address these problems. The way in which they may accept that burden might simply be at the local level in their community, where the underserved need to be the target of outreach and philanthropy; or it might be at the national or international level, where the underserved need to be a priority for policy initiatives. Either way, it is imperative for all physicians to integrate leadership into their practice at every level.

uplifting the medically underserved - I absolutely feel that access to a physician is a basic right. When Americans talk about life and liberty as human rights, as outlined in the Declaration of Independence, a big part of that is being healthy enough to enjoy life and liberty. So I think it kind of follows that if life and liberty are basic human rights, then access to treatment by a physician—regardless of financial ability—is something each individual is entitled to. Realistically speaking, not every country has the resources at this time to provide this guarantee to their citizens, but it is a goal worth working towards. Further, healthcare as a human right can mean much more than just enabling any person with medical concerns to see a physician. It can mean developing systems whereby the population as a whole is able to benefit from preventive care, cost-effective screening modalities,

and basic health education in both the school environment and throughout communities. Access to a physician is most optimal only in the context of a robust public health program.

a life apart - In any therapeutic alliance between a patient and physician, there is always this constant tension between our professional role as healer and our personal role as fellow human being. I don't think that tension in and of itself is a bad thing. If you feel any sort of conflict about how much emotion to inject into a patient interaction, then that shows you are being mindful of both professional and sentimental considerations. Trying to navigate that tension is one of the challenges of being a physician, but it is an incredibly important challenge to undertake. The emotional bond the physician helps to create can, in a lot of ways, define the patient's experience of receiving care. A lot of the best attending physicians I have worked with take time during rounds, with the entire team present, to converse with our patients and gain a little window into their personal lives. If time does not allow for that in the morning, they make sure to come back in the afternoon and catch up with the patient. Either way, even in a busy academic medical center, these attendings have made it a focal point of their practice to develop a relationship with the patient. I find this to be beneficial for multiple reasons—it increases patient satisfaction and physician satisfaction, it can improve the quality of care, but more importantly, it is just the right thing to do. If we did not invest any personal attention to the doctor-patient relationship, then it really is not much of a relationship, because it cannot be a one-way street. As much as the physical healing of the patient is the physician's primary goal, the process of healing must be done in a respectful and emotionally tactful way.

a story - One story I would like to share is of a man who I helped take care of on the general medicine service last year. He had a very debilitating syndrome called opsoclonus-myoclonus ataxia that had come on quite suddenly just a week or two prior to his admission: He had difficulty walking, was unable to use his hands to eat or write, and had trouble focusing his vision on anything because his eyes were fluttering all the time. On the first day of his admission, I could tell he was quite troubled with what was going on, as I imagine anyone who had suddenly lost almost all motor control would be. It was clear by the look in his eyes and the melancholy on his face that he was significantly distressed by his inability to do anything. He stayed on our service for about two weeks, during which time we tried a number of therapies for him, none of which seemed to help his clinical condition. Each morning during those two weeks, I would see him and ask him how he was doing, and each morning he would reply with enthusiasm, "Better!" When I conducted a neurologic exam, I would find that in terms of his mobility, he was unchanged compared to the day before, but he still insisted with utmost conviction that he was doing better. His unmitigated optimism was uplifting, and something I

found myself looking forward to experiencing every day. Through spending time talking to him during his stay, it became apparent that his entire outlook on his disease had indeed gotten much better. By the time he was discharged, even though his physical condition remained much the same as it did when he was admitted, he displayed such an inspiring level of graciousness and fortitude that it felt as though he was, in fact, a cured man. His exhaustive appreciativeness of the care provided to him by the entire team was so heart-warming that it was a powerful reminder about the effects a robust provider-patient relationship can have on the patient experience, as well as a great example of how we can derive as much inspiration from our patients as they can from us.

a lens into your life - For almost the last year, I have served as the student body president for my medical school. It has been an incredibly rewarding experience because it has given me an opportunity to work with my talented colleagues as well as our school's administration to advance initiatives that enhance the student experience. One of the things we have tried to focus on this year in the medical student government is opening the lines of communication between students, the administration, alumni, and current faculty to provide a more diverse range of mentorship opportunities for students. Mentorship is a passion of mine, because I think it can be difficult to develop both professionally and personally as a physician without some sort of mentor. A faculty mentor, who may or may not be in one's field of interest, can be a sounding board for ideas related to career aspirations, while simultaneously serving to promote emotional well-being. We have really tried to solidify the lines of mentorship within our medical school through a number of avenues. For example, students can now be linked directly with a alumnus in a field they are considering so that they have someone to communicate with in a zero-pressure type of environment. In addition, a "House" system has been developed here that connects students from every year in a longitudinal fashion so that students who are just starting medical school can seek counsel from more senior students. I think this model for advising allows for a lot more flexibility so that students can address their individualized mentorship needs, with the ultimate goal of accelerated personal and professional growth as a physician-in-training.

Made in the USA
Lexington, KY
29 July 2014